Also by Cortney Davis

The Body Flute (poetry)

Details of Flesh (poetry)

Between the Heartbeats:
Poetry and Prose by Nurses (co-editor)

I Knew a Woman

I Knew a Woman

The Experience of the Female Body

Cortney Davis

Random House · New York

All rights reserved under International and Pan-American Copyright Conventions. Published in the United States by Random House, Inc., New York, and simultaneously in Canada by Random House of Canada Limited, Toronto.

RANDOM HOUSE and colophon are registered trademarks of Random House, Inc.

Grateful acknowledgment is made to Doubleday, a division of Random House, Inc., for permission to reprint four lines from "I Knew a Woman" from *Collected Poems of Theodore Roethke*. Copyright © 1954 by Theodore Roethke. Reprinted by permission of Doubleday, a division of Random House, Inc.

Library of Congress Cataloging-in-Publication Data
Davis, Cortney.
   I knew a woman: the experience of the female body / Cortney Davis.
   p.   cm.
   Includes index.
   ISBN 0-375-50418-4
   1. Women—Health and hygiene—Case studies.   2. Women—Medical care—Case studies.   I. Title.
RA564.85 .D38   2001
613'.04244—dc21   00-045903

Random House website address: www.atrandom.com

Printed in the United States of America on acid-free paper

9 8 7 6 5 4 3 2

First Edition

Book design by Mercedes Everett

For Alexandra, Justine, Madisyn, and Nathaniel

I knew a woman lovely in her bones,

When small birds sighed, she would sigh back at them;

Ah, when she moved, she moved more ways than one:

The shapes a bright container can contain!

—*Theodore Roethke*

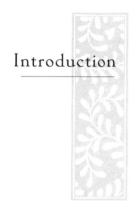

What happens to a woman in the privacy of a medical exam room has always been a secret between that patient and her caregiver. Although absolute knowledge of another woman's body is ultimately beyond anyone's reach, I have a critical advantage: the bodies of the patients I tend are like mine. As a nurse practitioner working in a busy OB-GYN clinic, I examine women daily, and I listen to the stories of their lives. Like them, I share the female body's bounty as well as its fluctuations, flaws, and undeniable path toward death.

Health care professionals, nurses as well as doctors, sometimes trivialize the field of women's health. During my first month in the clinic, I met a physician I knew in the coffee shop. When he heard what I was doing, he asked, "You *want* to work with women? Isn't it boring?" He wondered if I'd miss the "excitement" of medicine, as if thyroid storms and hormone imbalances and high-risk pregnancies were not dramatic. A nurse friend wrinkled her forehead and *tsk*ed, saying that she thought the maternity ward held little challenge. Didn't I prefer the stimulation of intensive care?

But when I came to work in women's health after many years as a nurse in critical care and as a nurse practitioner in specialty practices, I discovered a vibrant, provocative world. Unlike a psychiatric nurse or a college English professor, who must dwell for hours in the mind, I cannot ignore or move too far from the reality of the body, its glorious beginnings and its subtle endings. The regular beat of my heart is echoed in the pulse of hormones that bring on the menstrual cycle and also in the rhythm of my fingers as they palpate a patient's belly to delineate the organs beneath. I grasp all of evolution when I close my hand over an infant's head, deep in its mother's pelvis. I expose my own hidden places in the examining light that I shine on my patients' bodies. In the clinic, my patients and I are connected to the body histories and myths of all the women who have come before us and all those who will come after; together our experiences create the wider environment we call women's health.

This book tells the stories of four patients who struggle with the body's natural cycles as well as its unexpected surprises, and who, each in her own way, triumph. I write about Lila, Eleanor, Renée, and Joanna as an act of both rebellion and transformation: rebellion as I protest against the myopia of those who discount the importance of women's health; transformation as I acknowledge how caring for these patients has changed me. The details of their adversities and the determination with which they go forward humble and clarify my vision. There is a thin line between us women, between a nurse and her patient—perhaps only a day or a phone call between comfort and poverty, between health and disease. Between you and me in our kitchens with full cupboards and sizzling stoves, and Lila or Renée on the street. Between Eleanor in the operating room, and us safe in our beds. Between Joanna as she endeavors to make sense of the body's desires, and you and me as we adjust to the constant, primal tides that influence our lives.

As I wrote the stories of these women, I reviewed the narrative of my own life, if not always on the page, certainly in my heart. Like Eleanor and Joanna, I've experienced the body's disruptions. Like Renée, I've learned that the body and the soul can be at odds. Sometimes, often alone, we must wrestle with the flesh in order to allow the spirit to survive. Like Lila, I was, for a time, a welfare mother, struggling as a single parent without money, without a car, without a plan for the future. When I face my patients today, they see an educated woman whose situation might seem beyond their reach. But in their stories I see again where and how I was, and I remember that the path away from that place can be difficult to find and hard to travel.

The women's health clinic in which these stories take place is based in a suburban city hospital. It serves women from other countries without green cards or documentation, women and girls on welfare, the working poor, and those who have no insurance. For some of these women, the clinic becomes a haven, a surrogate family. There are nine rooms in the clinic, little cubicles that extend out from our narrow hallway like stubby arms on a lopsided octopus, three procedure rooms and six exam rooms. On the wall opposite the exam rooms, one of the nurses has put up a world map with little pearl-headed pins stuck into Ecuador, Mexico, India, Costa Rica, Chicago, New York City, and all the other places our patients come from. Inside each room, we've arranged an exam table with its hidden metal stirrups, a stainless-steel Mayo stand, a red-lined wastebasket for hazardous waste, and every instrument or supply any of us could ever need. We check the rooms daily in a ritual that's as soothing as making beds or doing laundry. We want the clinic to be clean and safe enough for our own mothers and daughters.

Some of us believe that women are better at caring for women than men are, and the smallest details of the clinic show this. The rooms may be small, but the walls are soft peach and curtains circle the exam tables in a billowy floral cascade. Inside this circle is a sacred space, a safe hideaway in which a woman can reveal what's on her mind. "I want to see a woman," many patients say, and the nurse writes "Female only" on the chart. Our male resident chuckles and stretches out his legs under the table. "Good," he says. "Less work for me."

There are eight residents in the clinic, three registered nurses, and me. The nurses and I work eight-hour shifts, five days a week. The residents are in the hospital almost all the time, covering the delivery room, the clinic, the emergency room, and the operating room, and taking call every third night. Each June two senior residents graduate, and every July two new, frightened interns arrive.

As a nurse practitioner, I fill a gap between the resident doctors and the nurses. I perform medical exams and procedures as well as nursing tasks. Like the physicians, I must sometimes inflict pain in the pursuit of healing, and I'm privy to the most intimate functions of patients' bodies. Like the nurses, I'm free to hug patients, to ruffle their hair and cajole them into little things such as enduring an exam or grand things such as trying to change their lives. Perhaps because I have, ultimately, less absolute power over illness than a doctor, patients are comfortable disagreeing with me, as well as telling me their secrets.

I'm also a poet, a caregiver who takes in another person's life through my eyes and my hands, then remembers it. When I write about patients, I'm caring for them in a complementary way, attending not only their bodies but also their souls. Writing about an individual patient makes her story forever a part of mine, and it helps me make sense of what happens to us as we go through our life cycles.

The stories in this book are based on true events, although the four central characters are composite portraits of many different women, and all of the details and the names and identification of patients, residents, physicians, nurses, and families have been disguised. I've also taken some liberties. Based on my clinical and personal intuition, I've occasionally imagined what examiners or patients might think or feel, and I've simplified medical explanations and treatments while staying true to the underlying facts. These pages are not intended to provide medical advice or to examine every issue in women's health, but to invite the reader to accompany me as I marvel at how women's bodies influence, and sometimes change, their lives.

What happens to a woman within the privacy of an exam room is crucially significant. That woman is our mother or sister, our wife or lover, our daughters, our granddaughters, ourselves. What happens to her happens to us all.

Author's Note

One of the great bonds between a patient and caregiver is that of confidentiality. In order to reveal herself physically and emotionally, a patient must trust that she will not be betrayed, that her story will not become gossip, bandied about or judged. Her story and her body are, after all, her most private possessions.

How, then, does a caregiver who is also a writer honor this trust? That question was of great concern to me as I wrote this book, and yet, like other nurses and doctors who write, I felt called upon to translate and pass on in some measure the extraordinary lessons I have learned from my patients' lives. I believe we become wiser, kinder individuals when we share another's suffering and recovery. I believe we are all curious on a deeply human level; our own lives become clearer and take on new shape when we listen to another's story.

Therefore, in the writing and revising of this narrative, I held fast to the emotional truths but let go the recognizable specifics of my patients' stories; their names, appearances, character traits, and even histories have all been altered and disguised to protect their privacy. In these pages, the only character represented factually is me, my thoughts and memories, my way of moving through the world of women's health. The patients in this book are all fictionalized composites, and my conversations with them have been created from my interactions with many women—patients and non-patients alike—the details replayed and reshaped. There is no one woman who could read this book and exclaim, "That's me!" Yet because the essence of women's experiences are, finally, quite similar, many women might read this book and recognize something of themselves.

I Knew a Woman

Chapter 1

*Dr. William Riley's office was five blocks from our suburban Con-*necticut home. It was 1962, several years before my mother would finally learn to drive, so she and I set off on foot, the form for my college physical folded in her pocketbook. Dr. Riley's office was the first floor of his home, a tidy two-story box just like the other wooden houses along Prosper Street—a name that surely reflected the aspirations of the town's founding fathers. A tinkling bell announced our arrival. Mother and I joined the handful of people waiting in straight-backed chairs around the edge of the room. Some patients were sniffling or coughing, others just stared at the floral carpet. Glass-front cabinets held a dusty array of fraying medical books, and the worn rugs and heavy curtains smelled like an old grandmother's apron. It was early summer.

In September, I would be a college woman. Almost eighteen, I was already convinced I knew more than my parents, certainly more than my mother. I had a boyfriend, and we'd had sex, an occasional slippery fumbling in the back of his Dodge that left me feeling powerful but not breathless and tingly. I was formulating a shaky theory: We women, I decided, had a magical, potent allure, as if we gave off some invisible chemical like the lovely nocturnal moths that cling to a screen door, driving the male moths mad. Men, for all their position in the world, were like these beating moths, humbled before us. Once a woman became a sexual being, I reasoned, she would always have the upper hand.

When my turn came, the doctor himself waved us in. He was short and partially bald, his few remaining hairs the color of old sand. Silver wire glasses sat halfway down his nose, and his cheeks were tight puffs of flesh, as if he held seeds inside or notes that he'd squirreled away in medical school for future reference.

I changed into my white gown (it smelled of Ivory detergent, and I imagined his wife as she washed a pile of gowns every day, holding her breath against whatever contagion clung to them), and Dr. Riley asked my mother the required questions about my immunizations and illnesses. Then he told her to sit in the wooden chair far across the room. As he examined me, I focused on Mother's thin, upright posture, her white gloves and unscuffed shoes, her splashy Lily shift aglow in the dim light. The doctor kept his blinds closed, creating a strange hermetically sealed dungeon, within which, I realized, a patient could lose orientation. I concentrated on my mother's bright image and the comforting hum of traffic outside the window, as if such human details could hold me to the real world.

I hadn't seen a line requesting "pelvic exam" on my college form, but Dr. Riley told my mother it was time to do one anyway. She nodded, and I suddenly wondered if he might discover I wasn't a virgin. Smug and well versed in street knowledge, I instantly planned to blame any lack of a proper hymen on horseback riding. Although I had no idea what a pelvic exam was, I assumed that once a woman experienced sex, she could endure anything. Mother sat, hands folded in her lap, and watched as the doctor extended the metal stirrups from his table and motioned me down. I was suddenly anxious about the exam and embarrassed by my mother's presence. Sitting to my left, she saw me slide to the end of the leather table, how the white paper stuck and bunched under me. Surely she saw how plaintively my bare knees stuck out, how the skimpy sheet was pushed back over my pubic hair. She saw the doctor bend slightly as he inserted first the metal speculum, then his fingers, into my vagina.

"She has a tipped uterus," he intoned to Mother, ignoring me as if I were simply the plastic model he used for demonstration. "I'll try to tip it forward again."

Mother nodded once more, asking something about difficult childbearing, and the doctor furrowed his brow. Small drops of sweat beaded in the waxy ruts of his forehead as he pushed another finger into me, wiggling it, leaning over until his cheek hovered above my pelvis. Once in a while he grunted something about my case being *difficult.*

This was before patients demanded explanations, before they asked questions, before there was any voice in the room other than the physician's. There was no nurse; my mother served as the only distant chaperone. She lowered her eyes and allowed the doctor to do what he thought best.

Dr. Riley continued twisting his fingers as he stroked my belly softly with his other hand, a mockery of the normal pelvic exam. I felt my limbs turn to stone. The control and the worldliness I felt with my boyfriend fell away like an old carapace I was forced to shed. "Hold still" was never said but certainly implied. The doctor in his white coat, my mother in her white pumps, the dark mahogany bookshelves and desk—everything in the quiet room whispered to me to be good, to endure. Outside was a different world: green buds unfurling, children in strollers. Me and my boyfriend, the car windows open and summer pouring in.

Ten minutes seemed like sixty, and I floated in time's unreal bubble. Surely what this doctor was doing was wrong, not the standard medical exam. I knew it, he knew it—*come on, someone speak up and tell him—enough!* When he finished, my insides throbbed and I thought my uterus must have burst. My inner thighs burned when I tried to stand.

Mother paid the bill (my poor mother, the obedient well-intentioned woman who would die at age seventy-eight, her last pelvic exam the one following my birth!), and we left, walked back down the tree-lined street to our white Colonial house with turquoise shutters, my college exam form folded in my pocket. I checked more than once, but nowhere did the words "tipped uterus" appear in the doctor's fountain pen scratchings. Nor did Mother and I talk about my exam. We only nodded in unison when she said, "I've heard that a tipped uterus makes it difficult for a woman to get pregnant. It's a good thing he could fix it."

Then I only suspected, but now I know. You can't rearrange a tipped uterus as if it were a piece of furniture in some tiny apartment. A "tipped" uterus is simply one of many variations of normal. Some uteruses are anteverted, curled over the cervix; some are midplane, extending straight out from the cervical neck; some are retroverted, tipped back beneath the cervix.

My encounter with Dr. Riley remained a foggy but persistent memory, like a book read and half remembered, until I was a student nurse practitioner learning to do pelvic exams in 1978. First we learned on hard plastic models, then on one another, then on patients.

"Here," the instructor said to me, "feel the uterus? Slide your fingers under the neck of the cervix and follow it until you feel the bulge of the fundus beneath. This uterus is retroverted." A nurse stood by the patient, one hand resting on the patient's arm. I had already explained the exam carefully and clearly, and after I inserted the speculum, the instructor and I positioned a mirror so the patient could view her own cervix. When I did the internal exam I didn't shove or wiggle my fingers, and I never said "Hold still." Then I felt it, the firm globular uterus, tipped back, like mine.

I caught my breath. The image of Dr. Riley, the light reflecting from his glasses and his moist forehead as he moved his fingers inside me, welled up in my mind's eye. Now I was the examiner, the one in control, yet I felt as vulnerable as I had that day in his office. I realized that I *knew,* viscerally and personally, how invasive this procedure is and how important it is that a woman trust her examiner. In the worst scenario, the exam room becomes the microcosm of a world in which a woman cannot be heard. In the best, the exam room is a privileged territory in which a woman learns how to be her own best advocate.

———————

Sometimes I wonder if Dr. Riley's exam was simply a distressing experience and not the misuse of power it seemed. After all, I do "first" pelvic exams almost every day, and I know how embarrassing and uncomfortable they can be. Or is it possible that Dr. Riley was trained to believe he could alter my pelvic anatomy, tip my uterus forward, and, as he said then, move my intestines to hold the uterus in place? Somewhere inside I want to believe that caregivers are above reproach, that none of us would dare take advantage of a patient.

But whenever I doubt my memories of that hot summer day, I remind myself of my final meeting with Dr. Riley. Right before I left for college, I developed a chest cold, and Mother suggested I go alone for a checkup. He took me into his exam room, told me to sit on that same massive old wood and metal table, and asked me to take off my shirt and bra. No drape or johnny coat this time. Still, no nurse. I sat with my young breasts pointing straight toward the buttons on his white lab coat, a line of small plastic disks that strained over the paunch of his belly as he leaned in to examine me. His stethoscope lingered on my breast, and I could feel his breath on my skin.

"You're a lucky young lady," he chuckled. "Look what you've got here." A touch, a brush of his finger as it circled my nipple. "Don't ever wear a bra, it'll ruin you." A squeeze of my thigh. A prescription for penicillin. Another squeeze.

———————

Again and again, I review my impressions of my visits to Dr. Riley, because those moments taught me a valuable lesson and they continue to influence my own practice in women's health. I try always to take care, explaining every step, draping my patients to preserve modesty, minimizing my touch and my movements unless that touch is a hug or a firm grasp of a patient's hand. I can never forget my own helplessness, so I don't lose patience with women who giggle inappropriately or cry out, who temporarily become too demanding or too frail. In Dr. Riley's musty office, I learned an emotional truth about the misuse of power and the importance of dignity and control, even for the youngest patient. Most of all, I'll never forget how swiftly and completely that first rush of self-esteem, that initial bounty of womanly grit, can be whisked away.

Chapter 2

Today, when I knock and walk into exam room 5, I find Lila, age fifteen, sitting on the edge of the exam table, fiddling with her sheet.

Right from the start, our positions are unequal. Lila is naked, covered with a blue-and-white flowered johnny coat and a sheet. She wears thick pink socks scrunched around her ankles and huge gold hoops that pull on her earlobes and hang down almost to her shoulders. "Lila" is spelled out along the side of the hoops in large gold letters.

I'm dressed in wool pants and a vest. My official white lab coat and the stethoscope draped around my neck proclaim my status just as surely as her nakedness announces hers. I've learned from the nurse's note that Lila is an emancipated minor, a girl whose parents or parent agreed to sign legal papers releasing her into her own custody. If Lila is a bad girl, if she's thrown out onto the street, if she wins the Pulitzer Prize, her parents don't want to hear about it. Sometimes parents have to emancipate their children. Tough love. Sometimes kids have to get away from violence, drugs, alcohol, or incest, knowing that nothing could be scarier than what they're already living. Sometimes good kids just get booted out. We may never know which story belongs to Lila. Before saying a word to her, before hearing a word she'll say to me, I'm already worried.

I've been a nurse practitioner for twenty years, longer than Lila has been alive, and I still can't get used to examining children. *Children.* The first time, years ago, it was a nine-year-old girl. Her skinny torso and gangly legs were far from womanly, but she had been attacked by her sister's friend and therefore thrust headlong into the sobering process of a rape investigation. I had to tend the jagged tear that split her labia. Under the light, her mons was hairless, smooth-skinned, and guileless.

As I worked, I was afraid I would hurt her more than she was injured already. Mostly, I was afraid that if something so horrible could happen to this girl, it could also happen to *my* daughter or *my* son. As I washed and dressed my patient's wound, I pictured my children. Their bodies, unlike hers, were still innocent and unaware. After the exam, the child's mother took me aside. "Is my daughter still a virgin?" she asked me.

In the clinic, I see young girls every day. Some are pregnant by accident or choice, some seek birth control or cure for infection, others worry about too-small breasts or irregular periods or finding someone to love. How, I wonder, can I help them retain their childhood and yet assist them to become women? How, I wonder, can I possibly help this Lila?

She's only a bit younger than I was when I had my first exam, so I touch her shoulder quickly in passing with a firm pressure meant to take away any sexual overtones yet offer reassurance. A motherly touch. Then I sit down on the round rolling stool in front of the exam table so we can talk. At least I won't be looming over her.

"Hi, Lila. I'm Cortney, a nurse practitioner here in the clinic. I'm going to do your exam today." It's my stock introduction, and, because she's so young, I give her more than my usual smile. Lila's face looks blank as a new sheet of paper. I'm grinning so hard my face hurts.

She doesn't look up, doesn't make eye contact.

"So, what can I do for you today?" I give her a few seconds. I know what she's probably here for—her annual Pap test, an infection check, birth control. But sometimes the answer to the question surprises me. Today, I figure my question might just get Lila to say *something.* She sighs and kicks her feet. I sit watching her while she stares at her socks.

"You know, I came for that test," she says, and begins to bounce one earring back and forth with a fingertip. As it sways violently, I worry that it might jettison from her earlobe.

"A Pap test?"

"Un-huh."

"So you're here for your annual exam."

"I guess."

"Good for you for coming in for it," I say, trying to be cheerful. In the back of my mind I review the rules. Women need annual Pap tests as soon as they are sexually active or by age eighteen even if they're not. I assume that Lila is sexually active, and I sense there's something else going on here too.

"Nobody likes this exam, but it's important. I don't like it either when it's my turn to be the patient."

That makes her smirk. But she doesn't look at me. I think she'll leave today not knowing who examined her.

"Lila, I'll start by asking you some questions about your health history."

She nods, and I go through the usual list of questions that begin "Have you had . . ." or "Do you . . ." or "When did you. . . ." I give her lots of time to think about the answers. Lila responds in grunts and nods, occasionally a two-word sentence. "Yes," she smokes a pack of cigarettes a day, she says, *"so?"* and "yes," she smokes pot once in a while and "yeah," she's done some coke, "who hasn't?" When I ask if she's had pelvic exams before she groans, "Oh yeah," but when I ask about abuse, she doesn't answer. When I talk about wanting to help if someone is hurting her, she looks interested in the variety of instruments laid out on the metal tray. When I offer an HIV screen, she coughs, and I wonder if she has reason to be nervous. The topic of birth control seems to perk her up, and she says that her boyfriend doesn't like condoms. I tell her that's what I hear from lots of girls, and Lila smiles a little for the second time.

Lila has had ten sexual partners but has never, she says, been pregnant. She doesn't know where her father lives—he won't tell her—and her mother has been out of the picture for years. Lila has tried to kill herself twice. She was in the hospital for three weeks after the last overdose.

Her boyfriend is twenty-eight, only seven years younger than her father, but Lila says that sex is consensual. Her father calls, tells her that he's going to have the boyfriend arrested, but Lila is emancipated and says she loves this man. She was living with a cousin, but they had a fight and the cousin threw her out. Now she lives with her boyfriend in his car.

She can't legally drop out of school until she's sixteen, but she rarely attends and the truant officers can't find her. She says she's looking for a job but hasn't found one.

Lila decides she wants to try the birth control pill, which she can't start taking until her next period. She thinks her last period was March 17. She doesn't want Depo-Provera, a birth control method delivered every twelve weeks by injection, because she hates needles, hates being hurt. We talk about that for a while, but we go in circles.

I study Lila carefully. She looks tough. At the same time, it seems as if everything about her has happened by accident. Her hair is dyed red, not the color I'd imagine her to choose, but red it is. Thin ragged bangs fan across her eyebrows, and the sides of her hair are ragged too. Lila's nose blooms with pimples, and her chin is so chapped I wonder if her boyfriend has a coarse beard. "Beard burn?" I almost ask but stop myself.

Lila's body is thin, painfully thin, with wing bones and knuckle bones and shin bones that stand out sharp and straight from her tight, pale skin. Her eyes are blue—not the clear blue of the chicory flower that will grow in my garden in June, more like the stain of fading ink. Her lips are ill defined and narrow. When I coax her into the vulnerable position women assume for a pelvic exam, I see that her legs are unshaven, the hair surprisingly dark and plentiful.

"This won't hurt," I say, trying to reassure her.

Her vagina is girlish. The smallest speculum is uncomfortable, and when I try to do the Pap test she slams her legs together, raises her bottom from the table as if I am forcing her to do something that reminds her of something she hates. I pause, chat with her, wait until her muscles relax and her buttocks loosen against the table and she seems ready. When I feel inside, tracing the size and shape of her uterus and ovaries, I can use only one finger. Her uterus is like a hard, tiny peach, and her ovaries are just a brief *ping* between my inside finger and my other hand on her belly. Lying down, she looks younger than she does sitting up.

When the exam is over, both Lila and I linger awhile, awkward and searching for an appropriate ending to this conversation. I give her sample packs of birth control pills. I give her written instructions on how to begin the pills with her next period. She doesn't look at me. Our talk, our dance of examiner and examined, must feel to her a little bit like love, a little bit like abuse. But I want Lila to trust that when she is in this room with me she is safe, a whole person who will not be judged. And so a graceful conclusion to this encounter is important, as important as a good last line is to a poem—a perfect line that, like a well-made door, closes the poem with a satisfying click.

Sometimes the last line needs an image or a simile. Lila slipping from the table like water. Lila bending over like the shadow of a hand. She dresses, pulls on another pair of socks and long johns, jeans, and two fraying sweaters. She looks for all the world like a drab, lost little girl as she walks out onto the busy street. Lila who lives in a car with a twenty-eight-year-old man. Lila who leaves her shoelaces untied and carries a backpack.

Chapter 3

What are women most afraid of when they come to be examined? Pain? Embarrassment? Learning that they have breast cancer or an abnormal Pap test? Patients like Lila—young, living foolishly on the edge of violence—sometimes I wonder if they have any fears. Most often, a woman's exam is normal, but women worry nevertheless. It's the older women, aware of how stubbornly the body rebels, who worry most. Eleanor McCabe, the forty-nine-year-old woman I see right after Lila on this cool late-March day, is more humbled by life and is the veteran of many exams. Few of my patients know the two things that scare me the most, but it will come to pass that Eleanor will find out about one of them.

"Hello," she says to me and extends her hand. "I'm Eleanor McCabe." She smiles, and I like her already.

In exam room 7, we talk awhile like friendly acquaintances, although I've never met her before. She's tall and broad-shouldered, her body just beginning to assume the vaguely lax outline of an older woman. Her frizzy brown hair is tamed with a short cut, and in the harsh clinic light, I see that her skin is finely lined, like tiny crinkles in just-washed silk. Sharp tucks deepen the corners of her eyes and mouth, as if she spends a lot of time in the sun. Her nose is big and bony, making her appear, oddly, both important and friendly.

When Eleanor's at ease—I can tell by the way her hands come to rest on her lap like large sleeping doves—I inquire about her medical history. We deal in particulars here: When did your periods start? How many days do you bleed? How many sexual partners do you have? How many pregnancies, how many deliveries? How were they, and what else has happened to you in your life?

I ask about personal habits (Do you smoke?), sexual preference (Do you have sex with men, women, or both?), and family illnesses (Have any women in your family had breast cancer? A heart attack?). Like a woman scrounging for change in the bottom of a pocketbook, I search out any secrets Eleanor's life might harbor. On the other hand, I rarely reveal anything about myself.

Her history is almost uneventful. Two of her children were delivered vaginally, the third by C-section. She had one miscarriage, a small tragedy in the middle of the night a long time ago. Her periods are regular, although at age forty-nine she's experiencing some perimenopausal symptoms. "My periods are heavier now," she tells me, and sometimes she passes blood clots—here she holds up her thumb and forefinger—the size of a fifty-cent piece. She chuckles when I ask about birth control. She had her tubes tied after her last delivery. "No more babies," she says, and her hands flutter up as if released by her laughter.

Eleanor answers my questions without hesitation. She knows that I'll soon see her naked, discovering what is beautiful about her body as well as what is not, and, like many patients, she warns me about her body's defects ahead of time, as if to ward off any possibility that I might be surprised or perhaps repelled.

"Oh, I hate the puckery skin on my thighs," she says. Then, "God, wait until you see this extra flab," as she points to her abdomen, making excuses for a belly stretched and marked by childbearing. But she knows that because I'm a woman, I'm like her. I, too, have bled through my jeans unexpectedly. I, too, am experiencing the body's slow changes.

When I ask about sexually transmitted diseases, Eleanor tells me she had genital warts when she was younger, a gift from her first husband. She knows a lot about the virus, how it lives in the body and can never be cured, but evidence of its presence—

annoying warts inside or outside the vagina, or an abnormal Pap test—can flare up whenever the body's immune system fails to suppress the viral activity. So far, she's been lucky. She's had an outbreak of the warts only twice. Both times, she had them removed from her labia with applications of acid. The wart virus can also occur on the cervix, but Eleanor tells me that as far as she knows, her Pap tests have always been normal.

When I inquire about sexuality issues, she says there's no problem, although once in a while, she whispers, she bleeds after sex or in between her normal periods, a light spotting that goes on for a day or two.

"I've also been having trouble sleeping. And I cry for no reason." Just telling me this, Eleanor's eyes fill, becoming bluer, and her nose reddens, accentuating the creases that slope down to her mouth and divide her face.

I ask if anything else is going on—marriage troubles, kid troubles? No, everything is fine. She likes her job as a part-time math teacher. She has a good marriage, although her husband recently lost his job. Now there isn't enough money and no medical coverage. "That's why I'm here in the clinic," she explains. I picture her sitting prim and proper in the crowded waiting room.

She says that before she lost her insurance, she'd related her symptoms to a medical doctor—the sleeplessness, the mood swings, the disturbing forgetfulness. She'd thought something was terribly wrong. He'd ordered a cardiogram, which had been negative, drawn some blood for tests, which had been fine, and then, since she didn't have anything "abnormal," he'd given her a small vial of tiny white pills for anxiety. "Just take it easy," he'd said. "And stop worrying." She'd walked out thinking she was crazy.

I tell Eleanor that women's symptoms are *different* from men's, that perimenopausal symptoms can really turn your world upside down. Odd dizziness, almost a vague off-balance feeling, as if the earth shifts once in a while, ever so slightly. The capricious monthly bleeding, sometimes on schedule, but then, for no reason, random or continuous. The skipped periods, the late periods, the headaches that occur a week before the bleeding begins. (Bleeding! Just the idea of bleeding every month, something women learn to

take for granted.) Hot flushes that begin after eating or in the middle of the night. The disappearance of dreams. A dense and dark
insomnia. Sleep disturbances that get worse during the full moon.
Perhaps most frightening, the cyclical unexplainable *pressure* that
some women feel, the arguments, the fear they will become too
angry. Memory loss, long before menopause or senility, as if tiny
black holes suddenly appeared in the mind's fabric, opening up so
that words or names or events could drop silently through. Then
the word coughed up, the rent in the fabric sewn shut, as if that de-
fect had never existed.

Once spoken, her confessions charge the air. I'm most worried
about Eleanor's irregular spotting. In a small portion of my brain,
I tick off the possibilities: infection, a cervical polyp, fibroids. Then,
two less likely diagnoses but ones that must be ruled out: endometrial cancer, cervical cancer. I tell her I'd like to do an endometrial
biopsy today after I do her Pap. By inserting a thin plastic catheter
into the uterus, I can obtain a small sampling of the uterine lining
and send it to pathology for evaluation. The procedure is crampy,
but it's over in a moment.

Eleanor says no, absolutely not today. She has an important faculty meeting to attend right after this appointment, and
she doesn't want to risk being uncomfortable. We agree that she'll
keep track of her bleeding pattern and come back soon to have the
biopsy. This discussion makes Eleanor a bit nervous, but another
part of her just as quickly dismisses any fears.

"Let's start with your neck," I say, and reach my fingers to trace
the chain of lymph nodes on either side.

As I examine Eleanor, I observe her. While she looks away, I
search for any tiny imperfections that might indicate illness, as
well as for those lovely human details: the few creamy flecks of
powder resting in the hollow above her collarbone; the freckled V
of skin still tan from last summer's sun, like an inverted arrow-
head. I place my stethoscope on her back, watching her skin expand and contract over her ribs as I listen to her lungs. Then I ask
her to lie back and raise her arms so I can listen to her heart and
examine her breasts. She tucks her hands beneath her head as if

she were merely lying on the beach, watching the seabirds glide overhead.

Eleanor's breasts are pendulous, and her areola are pink, the nipples large and prominent. When I was a student, I learned about the breast from *Gray's Anatomy,* a thick maroon tome with gold letters, long after I had discovered the breast's mythic powers in my own life. *Gray's* calls them "mammas," one letter away from Mama, and indeed, their primary function is the secretion of milk.

The breasts' earliest stirrings can be seen in an unborn six-week-old fetus, but the female breast truly comes to life during puberty, when the number of ducts and the amount of glandular tissue increase. More changes occur with each menstrual flow. Vessels engorge like a river's swollen tributaries, and the areola, the pigmented ring around the nipple, diffuses its stain like watercolor on porous paper. When I was eleven, I rejoiced at the first hint of puffiness, the soft way my nipple protruded a quarter of an inch beyond my flat rib cage. I longed for the time I would bend over and feel the delightful heaviness of my breasts as they responded to the pull of gravity, proof of their existence.

"Do you check your own breasts?" I ask Eleanor.

"Sort of. I check in the shower."

"Um-hum."

I examine her breast in segments, moving the tissue mass under my fingers like well-floured dough, beginning at the breast's outer corner, coming down and around clockwise. Every practitioner develops his or her own pattern. I've seen male residents wear gloves when they do a breast exam, believing that gloves decrease the sexual *feel* of this kind of touching, but I know that sex is in the mind as well as the fingers. The women residents and I use our bare hands.

"It's a good idea to check lying down, too. See how the breast tissue spreads out?" Her breasts are a typical combination of glandular and fatty tissue, thicker at the top and outer curve and smoother underneath the nipple. A firm ridge of tissue runs under both breasts, a common finding some women mistake for a tumor. Eleanor, like most women, has one breast that is slightly larger than the other. According to my *Gray's Anatomy,* it's usually the left, but in my experience it's just as often the right. In some women, one breast is significantly larger than the other. These women want to know what can be done. "Can I have an implant or a reduction on only one breast?" they ask, and I refer them to a plastic surgeon. In Eleanor's case, the difference is slight.

I compress her nipple, looking for discharge, and feel under her arm for lymph nodes.

"Do you feel comfortable doing your own exam?"

"Sure," she says. "It's just . . ."

"Scary, and hard to know what you're feeling."

I cover the left breast and expose the right.

"Yes," she says. "Exactly."

We talk about lumps that feel like stones or peas, lumps that are on only one side. Hard lumps, lumps that don't hurt, lumps that are painful. Lumps that swell before a period, then go down. I move Eleanor's breast under my fingertips, recalling the black-and-white drawings in the anatomy book: the breast cut in half showing the pendulous tissue suspended by Cooper's ligaments, the bands that slowly stretch, letting the mamma sag until, in ancient women, it is only a shriveled fold of skin.

"Your breast exam is normal," I say, sure of my diagnosis. There were no pebbly nodules hiding under the skin, no irregular areas that baffled me. Eleanor exhales and draws her johnny coat closed again. I'm also relieved. After her exam today, she'll have a mammogram, an X ray that compresses the breast between two Plexiglas plates, flattening the tissue like a dry sponge and bringing tears to the eyes. But good compression permits a clear X ray that can detect evidence of cancer several years before a woman might discover a tiny mass. The first time I had a mammogram, my knees almost buckled as the tech inched the plates down until the bulk of my breast was scarcely more than the thickness of my hand. Nevertheless, fearing cancer more than that temporary pain that stung like an attack of angry bees, I promised myself I'd return.

"It's time for the pelvic exam," I tell Eleanor.

I help as she places her heels into the open metal stirrups and slides her buttocks to the end of the table. *Like riding a bike.* Once you've learned this position, it's unforgettable.

"I hate this," she says, and, as I warm the speculum under running water, I agree. She pictures me naked on an exam table and feels better already.

I ask when she had her last Pap, and there's a six-beat hesitation.

"I was afraid you'd ask me that," she says. "I haven't had one in about five years."

I don't inquire, although perhaps I should, and she doesn't explain. Five years; way too long.

I sit on the rolling stool and slide to the end of the table between Eleanor's open legs. I'm wondering about her abnormal bleeding, her five years without a Pap test. I have no idea what I might find.

I drape the sheet around her thighs, then push back the middle to expose her vulva.

Chapter 4

I've never told anyone how different every woman's anatomy is, how the vulva can be plump or thin, the pubic bone high and ruffled with crisp hair or flat and silky. Or how the vaginal muscles sometimes contract involuntarily as I approach with the speculum, as if this delicate tissue can sense any alien presence, evidence of our vulnerability or perhaps a remnant of the skin's prehistoric memory of attack. I've never revealed how the sensitive flesh inside the vagina may be pink or bluish, or how, in a dark-skinned woman, the tissues can be a lush, surprising magenta.

I glance at Eleanor's face above the drape to see if she's ready, then place one hand on her knee.

"Let your legs relax open as far as you can."

This position is embarrassing, awkward, and degrading, and sometimes I say so. Today I say, "The more you can relax your legs and buttocks, the less discomfort you'll feel."

She lets her legs open, and the muscles of her inner thighs loosen, her buttocks flatten on the table.

I place the speculum against her leg. "Too warm?"

"No, it's fine," she answers. "Usually it's cold."

I move my other hand closer to her vagina.

"I'm going to touch on the outside first," I say, and proceed to examine the vulva, looking for warts, blisters, and early skin-color changes that might indicate cancer. Her labia are thin, evidence of waning estrogen, and her pubic hair, reddish interspersed with gray, is sparse.

I take two fingers and separate the labia, exposing Eleanor's pale vaginal mucosa.

"Here's the speculum," I say, and insert the blades vertically, turning them to a horizontal plane, a movement that must be done quickly, smoothly. I cringe when I watch students direct the speculum straight in, slowly, slowly, because they think a tentative advance doesn't hurt the patient as much. "Aim down, and move firmly but gently," I tell them.

Sometimes students learn on "pelvic models," women paid to act as patients. These experienced models are not at all shy about telling the nervous students what to do. "Not so much pressure there," they'll instruct. "No, move your inside hand to the left. You're trying to feel my ovary, not my stomach, for God's sake." First one student, then the next.

"Pressure," I say, and open the speculum blades until the cervix pops into view at the end of the vagina, looking like a smooth pink dome. When the speculum is introduced, and, a second later, when the blades are opened, it feels as if the vagina is being stuffed with terry cloth.

The small opening in the middle of the cervix is the os, the entrance of the canal that leads into the uterus. This canal is the narrow two-way path that permits the frantically swimming sperm to enter in search of the egg. Nine months later, it opens to welcome a baby, huge-headed and blinking, into our strange world of oxygen and bright lights. This is the passageway for the monthly blood, for the mucous discharge that lubricates and cleans the vagina.

Eleanor's cervix, after two vaginal deliveries, is large. I offer to hold a mirror for her so she can see too—something I often do to encourage women to understand their own anatomy—but she declines, laughs, and shakes her head. "No, thanks," she says. "I'll let you do the looking."

I inspect her cervix carefully for any evidence of abnormality, such as a benign polyp that might explain her bleeding or an erosion that might indicate a precancerous lesion, but I see none.

I pick up one sterile swab, direct it into the vagina, and place it into Eleanor's cervical os, letting it absorb any secretions that might reveal infection.

While I wait, we talk. She tells me she has no symptoms. I explain that chlamydia and gonorrhea may not give a woman symptoms, but if she has such a disease and it goes untreated, the bacteria may travel into her fallopian tubes, causing pain, fever, and, sometimes, infertility.

"That happened years ago to my friend," she tells me.

I remove the swab, place it in a special plastic tube, and snap off the end of the stick. Then I take a wooden spatula, a flat thin device like a Popsicle stick, and insert one end into the os.

"You'll feel some pressure as I do the Pap test, maybe some cramping in your abdomen." She gives a small sigh in agreement. I turn the spatula, collecting cells from the outside of the cervix, and smear the cells onto a glass slide. The uterus is a muscle, and like all good muscles it contracts when it's bothered, so both the culture and the Pap test cause a funny, hollow feeling of constriction in the pelvis. It feels, too, as if the vagina has tightened or perhaps been caught in a vise—not pain exactly, but the oddest pressure.

Next, I twirl the tip of a small brush in the os to scrape cells from inside the canal. As I do this, a drop of blood springs from the cervix. In a second, the drop of blood becomes a thin stream of red oozing into Eleanor's vagina.

"Your cervix is bleeding a bit from the Pap," I say. This is common in pregnancy and sometimes seen with infection or other problems. In my note, I'll write that she has a *friable* cervix—not so unusual, but something to be noted.

As I withdraw the speculum, I look carefully at the vaginal walls, so elastic they can stretch to accommodate a man's penis or a baby's head and so responsive they can clamp tight if a woman is afraid. Sometimes, particularly with a first exam, a woman is so tense her vagina closes like a door slammed in anger. The speculum cannot be inserted; even one finger is too intrusive.

Eleanor takes a deep breath, moves her legs. The labia resettle themselves around the vagina, the hairless inner lips again sheltering the canal. The next part, Eleanor knows, is not as uncomfortable.

"It's that clamp I hate," she says.

"Every time I do an exam I try to figure out a better method, but I haven't come up with one yet."

Eleanor laughs, a contagious chuckle.

"That's why I like a woman doing this," she says, lifting her head off the table to look at me. "You know what it's like."

I open a silvery foil packet of lubricant, cover the two first fingers of my right hand.

"This will be cold," I say, and separate the labia with my thumb and fourth finger, slipping in my index and middle fingers. The vagina closes around them, and the lubricant warms. I reach deep to the cervix. It feels firm and rubbery, like the tip of a nose. Sometimes, especially when we fit diaphragms, we teach women to feel their own cervixes. They're always surprised at the unexpected resistance.

I put pressure on the cervix, move it back and forth. The uterus and ovaries shift with it, but Eleanor stares up at the ceiling with no indication of discomfort. Then, keeping two fingers under the cervix, I bring my other hand to her abdomen.

"Make your belly as soft as you can." As she relaxes, I trap the sphere of the uterus between my inside fingers and my outside hand. While Lila's uterus felt like a small peach, Eleanor's is a large lemon, slightly bulky after her three pregnancies and anteflexed, curled up over her cervix.

"Does this hurt?" I ask, tracing the outline of her uterus.

"No," Eleanor says. "Just feels like I'm being examined."

I slide my fingers to the left of the cervix and press my hand on the right side of her belly, feeling for her right ovary. It slips over my inner fingers, a little *blip,* like a peeled grape. Eleanor winces.

"That discomfort is normal," I reassure her. I reverse the procedure for the other side. Again, the fleshy grape, the twinge of pain.

"All finished," I say, and she lifts herself back into a sitting position. "I don't find anything obvious that might be causing the spotting. There are no cervical polyps, and your uterus and ovaries feel normal. No evidence of fibroids or a cyst." I don't say that an early endometrial cancer might cause spotting—although the risk of that is less than 10 percent—or that an abnormal Pap is possible even with the most benign-looking cervix. I don't say that what's going on with Eleanor is a bit of a mystery. Her symptoms might simply be perimenopausal, an uncomfortable constellation of signs that occur as her estrogen production begins to wane. I could tick these common problems off to her, one-two-three, dismiss them as "nuisance symptoms" that might be dulled by a low-dose birth control pill. But Eleanor, like other perimenopausal women, might not consider these events a mere nuisance. To her, unpredictable spotting, insomnia, and a vague depression might make the difference between a day lived and a day simply tolerated.

After she dresses, we discuss the options. Until we know why Eleanor is spotting between her normal periods—an occurrence that, in a perimenopausal or postmenopausal woman, must be considered an indication of cancer until proven otherwise—I can't give her any medication. Instead, she and I have more work to do.

"I want to know more about what you're experiencing. Then we can figure out what might help." I ask her to keep track of her symptoms and her irregular bleeding. It will help us both to know which symptoms are the most annoying and when they occur. Also, what I discovered today about Eleanor through my eyes and my hands provides only part of the evidence. In the old-fashioned "medical model" of communication, where the caregiver asks the questions and then makes his or her pronouncements, mine would be the loudest voice in the room and I would be the one with all the answers. But to me, what a patient thinks, feels, and says is primary. The real clues, the missing pieces of the puzzle, must come from Eleanor.

I ask her to return for the endometrial biopsy and promise that she will be called right away if there are any problems with her Pap smear or cultures. Before she leaves, Eleanor shakes my hand.

"Thanks so much," she says, smiling, "for being kind."

Of course, not all exams are easy, and not all patients are like Eleanor. "What about the really awful patients?" my friends ask. "How can you do *their* exams?" But, a good nurse, I don't reveal everything. I shrug my shoulders and tell them it's a job, like any job. I don't tell them the real truth—that nothing about the body disgusts me. It's what's *in* the bodies that gets to me: the diseases; the bent and broken souls.

Chapter 5

Outside, dusk has arrived. The air is cold and blustery, and I'm tired, anxious to get home. It has been a long day of new patients, and here is one more. Joanna, the young woman in exam room 3, has the last appointment today, the one day a week I work the evening clinic.

"I have this horrible pain inside," she says. She jabs her finger at her lower abdomen. "I think maybe I'm allergic to sex."

I lean back on my rolling stool and look up at her. She's in her early thirties, sitting fully dressed and poised at the end of the exam table. What she says seems almost humorous, not at all what I'd expect from someone in pain. In response to the confused tilt of my head, she smiles.

When Joanna made this appointment, she told the secretary she needed to find a GYN provider, something she'd been meaning to take care of since she moved here from Manhattan. She wasn't due for a Pap test, but she wanted an appointment anyway, she said, to be "checked." Her hair is walnut brown, short and tapered back only at the sides. As she runs her hands though it, waiting for my response, it falls perfectly into place. She wears eyeglasses with thin black frames, and she's dressed all in black: straight-leg pants and a zip-front sweater, stockings and leather shoes. No makeup, I notice, except for maroon lipstick that makes her teeth look startlingly white. She has maroon nail polish on, too. A silver pendant hangs from her neck on a long chain, swinging whenever she leans forward.

Patients who come in for visits in the evening are, for the most part, working women without health insurance. Sometimes they are women who, in spite of full-time employment, can't afford a car or rent. Other times they are like Joanna, educated, middle class, but nevertheless uninsured. Because, like me, these women can't take time off from their jobs for routine but necessary matters such as annual exams, we try to accommodate them. Once a week, I come into work around lunchtime and stay until eight. Unlike the day patients, who are seen by whoever picks up their charts, the evening patients are scheduled to see me specifically. From four-thirty to seven, patients arrive every half hour. They sit in the waiting room reading novels or flipping through magazines.

I like my evening clinic. All the residents and nurses and secretaries are gone, and the phones are rolled over to the answering service. Everything is slower and quieter, and the darkness outside seems to enhance the sense of intimacy. Because my assistant is a nurse's aide, by law not allowed to give instructions to patients, I must do the teaching that the registered nurses do during the day. I get to spend more time with patients, an opportunity to listen without interruption and so better address their concerns: how the various types of birth control work, how labor progresses into delivery, the benefits and risks of hormone replacement therapy. I also see new patients, such as Joanna, in the evening. Because we've never met before, she and I have that odd potential that anonymity affords—the freedom to get into things we might be shy about if we knew each other better, or if there were a crowd of other patients buzzing around outside our door.

Although patients often don't tell the secretary or the nurse the *real* reason for their visits, Joanna's statement—her response to my question "And what can I do for you tonight?"—takes me by surprise.

"Why do you think you're allergic to sex?" I ask. I'm not sure what else to say.

"Because every time I have intercourse, I get this terrible pain."

"Tell me about it."

"It starts here," she says, gesturing in the midline under her pubic bone, "and it ends here." She points to a spot under her umbilicus. Although Joanna continues to smile, her movements are sharp, as if they alone might acknowledge her discomfort.

"When do you think the pain is worse? When your partner first enters or during intercourse?"

She slips her hands under her thighs, and her posture changes to that of a demure little girl. At first I think she may be embarrassed by my question, as some women are. But unlike those women, Joanna's answer is explicit, almost technical, and her voice doesn't waver, a sharp contrast to her timid pose.

"Basically, it hurts all the time," she says. "When David enters me, when he moves, when he withdraws. After, my vagina burns for hours, and sometimes my abdomen aches until the next day."

"How long has this been going on?" I ask, and Joanna doesn't hesitate. "For months," she says. "And it's getting worse."

Pain with intercourse: it's one of the most frequent complaints we hear in the clinic, as well as one of the most frustrating to decipher. There are so many possible diagnoses, and the hunt to track down the pain's source can be long and involved, distressing for both patient and caregiver. Once in a while the answer is straightforward. Sometimes a uterus that is retroverted, or flexed back behind the cervix, can cause discomfort during sex. Jarred by the penis, the tipped-back womb rocks and pulls; the pain stops after intercourse but sometimes leaves a dull ache deep in a woman's pelvis for several hours, a common problem that might be corrected by altering the sexual position to allow the woman to control the depth and angle of penetration. Or a woman might have a urinary tract infection, a vaginal infection that requires antibiotics, or a small ovarian cyst that will go away on its own. More often, there's no simple answer.

"Is David a recent partner, Joanna?" Sometimes unexpected symptoms occur with a change in relationship—the effects of different lovemaking techniques, tension, infection, or even chemical irritation as a woman's vaginal environment responds to the new man.

"No," she says. Her smile is fixed, and she holds her shoulders hunched up and her hands pinned down, as if she were trying to keep herself still. It appears to me that if Joanna let down her guard, she might agitate off the table or leap up and pace the room. For a moment, I wonder if I should mention this to her. I could say, "You're smiling, Joanna, yet to me you seem very anxious."

"I've been with David for several years. Sort of unofficially engaged. I moved in with him about six months ago," she adds.

"Have you noticed anything else? A change in your vaginal discharge or pain at other times?"

She takes one hand from under her thigh and points at her pelvis again. "It feels like there's something swollen in there," she says. "Sometimes when I look down, it seems like one side of my abdomen is bigger than the other."

This is an unusual symptom, so I become a bit more alert. Often women complain of bloating, particularly before a period, and many times women worry about increasing abdominal girth, which can be one of the early warning signs of ovarian cancer. But unilateral swelling? I try to keep an open mind.

"You said the pain is getting worse."

"Worse every time we have sex. I hope you can help me," she says.

Polite, I think, trying to read Joanna's signals. No, not polite. Stiff. Afraid. Her words are explicit and articulate, but her body language tells me something else. It tells me that Joanna is not only nervous, she's also completely humiliated. Walking into the room, I had instantly and incorrectly assumed that her sophisticated appearance meant that she was well educated about her body and would be easily conversant about such intimacies.

"So," I recap, smiling back at her and softening my voice, "you have pain that occurs with sex and continues to ache afterward. And you have vaginal burning. Does that also persist after intercourse?"

"Yes," she says.

Spontaneously, I reach over to touch her knee in a gesture of reassurance but, catching myself, draw back. I'm not sure Joanna would welcome such physical contact.

"Pelvic pain is a very common problem, something I hear about a lot," I say. "We'll figure it out."

She raises her eyebrows, and two streaks of color, maroon like her lipstick, appear on her cheeks. Her face is small, heart-shaped.

"Do you have this pain or burning at any other time?" I ask, trying to organize her symptoms into a logical constellation and line up possible diagnoses. Caregivers and patients both believe that if we can actually assign a name to symptoms, we can also fix them, box them up and ship them out for repair. Truly understanding what any patient tells me is the challenge. Will she and I agree that I've "got it," that I can both intellectualize and empathize with what she's experiencing? With Joanna, one question at a time, I try to rule out urinary tract infection, endometriosis, even a pulled muscle.

"Do you have burning when you urinate?" I ask. Sometimes, with other patients, I have to say "when you pee?" Joanna says no. "Do you experience this same pain with your periods, with bowel movements, or randomly?"

Again, she says no. "How about with physical activity? Does walking or changing position bring on the pain?"

"No," she says. "I never have it at any other time. Only with sex."

"Does the pain go away or get better if you and David change your position during intercourse?"

"No, it doesn't make any difference. It *always* hurts."

I take a quick look at the wall clock. Part of me still hopes we might arrive at some simple solution. It's quarter after seven. Usually, I relax and enjoy the late hours with patients. Other evenings, such as tonight, I find myself torn between my dual roles, caregiver at work and caregiver at home. I want to learn more about Joanna, and I want to make her comfortable, at ease. But I'm beginning to feel filled up, like a jar that can hold only so much water. She responds to my questions quickly but not generously. I ask a question; she gives me one small fact. Every bit of information I elicit is like an added drop. Drop by drop, the meniscus rises, quavering and about to spill over.

She's a college graduate and a freelance graphic designer who works for herself after four years as an employee in large advertising firms. She has always been healthy: no illnesses, no operations, no tobacco or drug use. She drinks wine only on social occasions. She hasn't had any other sexual partners since being with David. She's sure he's faithful, as she is. When I ask, she tells me she had three other partners before him, one at a time in fairly long-term relationships, what we call serial monogamy. Her first sexual experience was at age twenty, later than for most of the patients I see here in the clinic. I ask if she has ever been pregnant, if she has had any sexually transmitted diseases or abnormal Pap tests in the past, and what about birth control? She's never had any STDs, she says, although she has had an occasional yeast infection. No, no abnormal Paps, and she has never been pregnant. She's on the pill and takes it faithfully. She has no other symptoms. Her appetite is great, she says. In spite of the current *pain issue,* she tells me, her relationship with David is good.

"Have you ever been sexually or emotionally abused?" I ask, and she looks at me as if trying to recall. Her gaze is direct but not open. No, she shakes her head, and the layers of her hair sway. No. She's never had *any* problems. That's why she can't understand these symptoms, this weird swelling.

I tell her I'll do a limited exam targeted at uncovering the possible reasons for her vaginal burning and pelvic pain. She agrees to obtain her records from her previous gynecologist, then come back to follow up on whatever we find, or don't find, tonight. I wait in the hallway while Joanna undresses.

When I return, she's already stretched flat on the table, the sheet hardly covering her. I'm surprised and somewhat disconcerted to find her this way. Usually, a patient waits until I pull out the footrest, and even then I often have to coax her to lie back— nobody likes this exam. But Joanna has flaunted the unspoken routine, and her immodesty is in startling contrast to what I previously perceived as embarrassment. I feel, more than usual, the impact of examining a stranger's body, a discovery I repeat several times a day with different patients, each time with the same sense of privilege and responsibility. But with Joanna, I sense that I must take extra care. Her signals may be disconcerting to me, but mine must not confuse her.

I open the sheet fully to cover Joanna, then fold back the top. I talk to her as my fingers trace the curve under her jaw and the hollows behind her clavicle bone. I tuck my stethoscope beneath her breast and count her heartbeats, listening to the way the valves open and close in sequence and how the blood rushes through the leaflets. I hear how nervous she is, her heart pumping full, individual throbs that make a visible pulse in the fleshy space between her breasts where the silver pendant nestles. I probe the convexities of her abdomen and learn her secrets. She has a line of downy auburn hair running up from pubis to umbilicus. The small tether of the umbilicus, where she was plucked and cut free from her mother, protrudes out in a pale knob. I thought her skin would stretch tight between her hipbones, but instead I find that it creates a soft purse, a tiny belly.

All this, the laying on of hands—something that nonmedical people rarely experience or think about. I remember what a friend told me after her first day as a volunteer in the emergency room. For her initial assignment, she had to help dress an elderly man. In the process, she lifted his bare foot, trying to work a sock over his heel. Curious and moved by this unfamiliar contact, she wrapped her fingers around his arch, around his toes, and held his foot for a moment, warming it. This simple act, she told me, transformed her—the roughness of his skin against hers, his bony joints, his calluses and prominent blue veins. There was *her,* and then there was this *other.* Before that, she had known only her husband's body, her children's. Family. And you, she said to me, you touch patients in the most intimate places, as if it were nothing.

"No," I replied, "not as if it were nothing." Their nakedness and my touch: the great equalizer.

———————————

Before going on to the pelvic exam, I hesitate a moment.

"All set, Joanna? If you'll just slide to the end of the table and put your heels in the stirrups." I pull them out, and Joanna inches herself down. I swing the light around, then turn to the sink, pull on my gloves, and hold the speculum under warm running water. My assistant has set up a cervical culture, which I'll use to rule out chlamydia and gonorrhea. I take out slides to do a wet mount as well, a microscopic exam to check for yeast, bacterial vaginosis, and trichomoniasis, common infections that might cause discomfort or irritation. Because of Joanna's symptoms, I anticipate a difficult exam. I expect Joanna's muscles will involuntarily tense, her knees refuse to separate.

Yet as I proceed, Joanna simply lies there, permitting me to examine her as if she feels nothing. She turns her head to the side and stares at the patterned curtain surrounding the exam table. Like a mime, frozen in her pose before passersby, Joanna doesn't twitch a muscle.

The sensitive skin around her vulva is irritated, slightly red, as if she'd scrubbed the area with harsh soap. When I touch her, I expect her to flinch, but she barely takes in a breath. Inside, her vaginal walls appear healthy and pink with the usual amount of clear, odorless vaginal discharge. Her cervix, too, is pink, small because she is childless and with a pinpoint os. After taking the cultures, I examine her uterus and ovaries. I ask, "Does this cause the same pain you experience with intercourse?" but Joanna remains silent, motionless.

"Your uterus is here," I say, outlining the small, anteverted oval and watching her face. "Totally normal."

I palpate her ovaries, one slightly fuller than the other, not an unusual finding. Neither ovary is enlarged or tender. Before I withdraw my examining hand, I turn my fingers over and sweep the floor of the vagina, feeling for the cobbled nodularity that sometimes occurs with endometriosis, but there is nothing.

"I don't feel any cysts on your ovaries," I say. Again I ask, "Did the exam cause you any pain?"

"No," Joanna replies, and she pulls herself up to a sitting position.

I tell her I'll go examine the slides under the microscope while she dresses. Then we can talk. When I return, I find Joanna standing in front of the table, still partially undressed and holding the sheet so it covers her pubic hair and exposes her belly. Immodest and remarkably detached, yet at the same time childishly vulnerable.

"Do you see what I mean about swelling?" she asks. "See how the left side sticks out more than the right?"

I try to visualize what Joanna sees but notice nothing out of the ordinary. The abdomen is never totally symmetric, and the contour might be altered by a woman's posture, by stool moving through the large intestine, by the bloating that occurs around menstruation or after a meal.

"Right now," I say, "your abdomen looks totally normal."

Knowing that we're *normal* is all most women want. We can tolerate just about any symptom, any strange occurrence, if we know that it falls within the realm of "what's expected." When women point out their physical oddities to me—one larger breast, an inverted nipple, labia that seem too prominent—they ask, "Have you ever seen this before?" When a woman has breast tenderness or pain that lances through her abdomen in between periods, sometimes she says, "I can stand it as long as I know it's normal."

"I'm not sure anymore *what* normal is," Joanna answers. "I just know there's something in there that's causing me pain."

I motion for Joanna to sit down. She raises the sheet to her shoulders, tenting her body.

"Your exam is completely fine," I say. "I didn't find any evidence of infection under the microscope. Your ovaries and uterus," I repeat, "are normal size and shape."

I might attempt to place my hand on her arm to comfort her, but she has made the sheet into a barrier, warding off any physical connection. I can't make out the contour of her arms or legs beneath the white expanse.

"Joanna, I have a few ideas about what might be going on. I'll send the cultures to the lab to rule out any serious infections. In the meantime, we could look at some other options. Are you willing to try a few things and then come back?"

"OK," she says.

"It's possible that the vaginal irritation and the pelvic pain may be related. If the vagina is dry, not sufficiently lubricated prior to sex, intercourse can be painful. Once that happens a few times, you anticipate the pain and the problem is perpetuated. Sometimes couples don't allow enough time for foreplay. Sometimes, if there's a problem in the relationship, it's difficult for a woman even to consider being sexual."

Often, this is where a patient interrupts me. "Yes," she might say, "you know, I just don't seem to get excited anymore." Or she might say, "Well, things aren't so good right now. I only have sex because he wants to. It hurts so much I could do without it." I'm curious about what might have changed in their relationship since Joanna moved in with David, but she volunteers nothing.

"You might also try using a really mild soap and washing the vaginal area only once a day, gently. And it's not a good idea to douche. That can upset the natural balance inside the vagina and cause irritation."

"I'll try changing soaps," she says. "I never douche anyway."

"It would help me if you kept a pain record. Take a pocket calendar and mark down when you have your period, when you have intercourse, and when you have the pelvic pain. Sometimes it's easier to find a correlation that way."

"I can do that," she says. "So I guess I'll finish getting dressed."

She stands, as if she's decided that this is where the visit ends. I stand, too, and push my rolling stool into the corner. For a moment, I'm worried that she might have seen me before, glancing at the clock.

"When do you want me to come back?" she asks.

"In six to eight weeks. That will give us enough time to see if there's a pattern to the pain. But if you think the pain is increasing or something else develops, please call me sooner."

"And here," I add, handing her some silver packets of lubricant, the same water-soluble jelly I used for the pelvic exam. "Try using this when you have intercourse. It will provide some lubrication and minimize the irritation."

"Thank you," Joanna says, smiling. The parting is pleasant enough, but I feel as though she and I have spent the visit talking in two separate rooms.

As I drive home, I can't stop replaying my visit with Joanna. Her apparent emotional isolation and her passivity during the pelvic exam concern me as much as tears would have. Involuntarily, I shiver. I'm not a mind reader. I can't guess what she's not able to reveal, but certainly there is *something* lodged inside Joanna that's causing her pain. What I want most is to stop thinking about her. I'd like to shed today's sights and sounds and go home to my house and my husband without other women's problems trailing from my fingertips like ragged seaweed. I visualize myself plunging into a peaceful lagoon. I pretend that when I emerge, my memory of the day will be washed away. All the faces of all the women will disappear, wiped from the slate of my mind as easily as my grand-daughter's words are lifted from her Etch-A-Sketch.

Instead of hurrying to make dinner, I pick up a pizza. Then I take a long shower, giving myself an hour to readjust to my own rhythms. Don't we say this every day in the clinic—that we women value service to others but often don't find the time to nurture ourselves? As I step into the cascade of hot water and steam, I banish Lila, Eleanor, and Joanna from my mind.

Chapter 6

It's late May when Lila's name pops up again, this time on the list of patients coming in for their first pregnancy visit. I'm surprised and then disappointed. I guess she never started that pack of birth control pills I gave her—when was it, back in March? I wonder if the father of this baby is Lila's twenty-eight-year-old lover, her living-in-a-car boyfriend. I wonder if Lila has ever had any good luck.

Thursdays from noon to five we see pregnant women at high risk because of other problems: women with diabetes, women carrying twins or triplets, women who are drug-addicted or in the methadone program, women who have high blood pressure or problems with their platelets or that catchall problem, "poor social circumstances." Women over thirty-five are at greater risk of having babies with birth defects. So are teenagers, a susceptible group with an increased chance of premature deliveries and fetal deaths. Our oldest pregnant patient is forty-seven. Our youngest is twelve, although we once had a ten-year-old.

Outside the clinic, the hospital ground crew is busy with fertilizer and rakes, and the dirty, half-melted snow has disappeared into the earth. After Memorial Day, the hospital gardens will erupt into yellow and pink and I'll go for walks in the nearby cemetery at lunch, but right now all I want to do is go home and sit on my porch. Today, I tell myself, I'm too overcome with spring fever to deal with Lila, maybe somewhat reluctant to face her as well. Why couldn't I reach her the first time I saw her?

When I walk into the room, Lila exclaims, "Oh hi, it's you." I figure I've gotten a standing ovation.

"Remember me?" she asks.

"Sure I do. How are you, Lila?" Next comes the part I hate. Hate and like.

Lila grins, the biggest grin I think she's capable of, and she says, "I'm pregnant. Great, right?"

Right. On one hand, I love how some women cry the first time they hear the gallop of their babies' hearts and how a patient might give up her bad habits, smoking or drinking, just like that, for the sake of her unborn. I like to watch women's bellies expand week by week until I can trace the outline of their babies for them and they can imagine the small fingers and toes. On the other hand, I've seen too many teenagers who think pregnancy is a diversion, like playing with dolls. Their growing bellies slow these young mothers down and dull their spirits. When their babies arrive, naked and imperfect, they demand too much. Banished out of sight, the babies doze in their carry seats in front of the TV, their bottles propped up so they can drink.

It's chilly in the clinic, the air conditioner recently stirred to life by the rising humidity, and Lila's legs are stippled with goose bumps. Her right eye is ringed by a dull greenish-purple bruise, and I see a meaty red patch on her cheek where the flesh has been skinned away. When the nurse handed me Lila's chart, she whispered, "Looks like someone beat her up."

"I got a room with my girlfriend now," Lila says, and she actually looks at me.

"Wonderful, no more living in the car!" I *am* relieved to hear that. I ask how her boyfriend feels about her pregnancy.

"He's really happy too. He has a boy already, so he hopes this one is a girl. If it's a girl I'll call her Tiffany Leigh."

"Tiffany. That's a nice name, Lila." I wait, a small pause. "Your boyfriend has another child?"

"Yeah. Tyler. He's, like, three." Lila pushes her red hair out of her eye. I notice, with a small sense of loss, that her gaudy hoop earrings are gone, replaced by crystal studs the color of pistachio ice cream—Lila's nod, I decide, to the warmth in the air. A time of planting and flowers blooming. Lila, I realize, is aglow with love and longing.

Her plan, she says, is to save money and get an apartment with her boyfriend, whose name is Charles. When I ask where he is now, Lila's face goes blank again, and, as quickly as that, she avoids my eyes.

"He's living at home with his mom"—and, I find out, with his son, Tyler, and Tyler's mother, his old girlfriend. Charles's mother thinks Lila is white trash. When she found out Lila was pregnant, she invited her son to come in from the car. His first girlfriend and Tyler moved in, too, and they banded together to convince Charles to dump Lila. He dropped Lila off at the city shelter. But that shelter didn't take pregnant women, so Lila, summoning what energy she could, went to Family Services and hooked up with a social worker. The social worker found another teenager who lived in a two-room apartment above a restaurant. Lila moved in, and she liked the other girl at once.

Charles occasionally comes over to sleep with Lila, and she figures he's sleeping with Tyler's mom as well. On her OB form, I see that Lila has checked yes to question number fifteen: "Is the father of the baby involved?" And yes to number sixteen: "Are there others who will be supportive?" Lila is building a make-believe family.

I recall Lila's health history fairly well, but we review it again. Yes, she groans, her last period was March 17, and it was normal.

"Remember?" she asks. "I saw you when I was almost due for my next period, but it never came." I nod.

"So you missed your period in April. That would make you about . . ." I turn my pregnancy wheel. I point the "Last menstrual period" arrow to March 17, and the "Expected delivery date" arrow falls on December 22. "About ten weeks pregnant today with a due date of December 22. In a few weeks we'll do an ultrasound, and that will tell us exactly where you are. Then we can pin down a due date for sure."

I look up. Lila is studying her lap. "Christmas," she says.

"Maybe. That would be nice." I try hard to sound enthusiastic.

I recall that Lila has a history of depression and suicide attempts, that she has a long history of abuse, and that she has been, off and on, homeless. She is a heavy smoker, and she has dabbled in drugs. She has minimal contact with her father and none with her mother, and her boyfriend's certainly not a reliable source of support. She's fifteen, just, and she won't turn sixteen until after the baby's born.

What I want to do is to shake Lila, shout at her, "What the hell are you doing?" Instead, I ask, "Are you sure, in your heart and in your mind, that having a baby now is what *you* want?" The question hangs there, turning slowly in the air like the paper mobile suspended above the exam table.

I have asked this casually, routinely, but Lila looks horrified and more than a little angry.

"What, you telling me I should have an abortion or give my baby up?"

"I'm asking to make sure that *you* want this baby and that you're not having it because you think your boyfriend will love you more if you do, or because he told you he wants a baby, or because you think if you have his baby he'll leave Tyler's mom and come back to you."

"I don't give a shit what he does," she says. "It's my baby." Lila raises her chin and looks as if she has just aged about five years. I feel myself aging too.

"OK, Lila. We have a social worker. She's here to help with housing, money, child care, whatever you might want. There's a teen mentoring program too." I can tell by Lila's glazed look that I've lost her. I make a note on her chart to have Meg see Lila on the next visit. Then we get on with the exam.

Lila's ribs make ridges in her back that my fingers climb like a ladder. I listen to her heart thudding, betraying her anxiety. I see a rosy blush dot her cheeks.

"Jesus," she says as I examine her breasts. "Don't kill me."

Lila rolls her eyes. I figure all this negative feedback means we're bonding.

Her abdomen is still flat and as hard as the expression on her face. In my mind, I see her belly expanding, growing with the ever-moving fetus underneath. I wonder if Lila has any idea what she's in for. I point out the faint line just beginning to trace its way from her belly button to her pubis. *"Linea nigra,"* I say, the calling card of pregnancy, caused by hormonal stimulation of the skin's mela-nocytes, the pigment-producing cells. Destined to fade after deliv-ery, it leaves its imprint on the abdomen forever. Lila raises her head to look. Her nipples, she points out, are turning the same shade of brown. As the weeks go by, her breasts will increase in size. Blue feathery veins will appear under the skin's surface, lac-ing the alveoli like a delicate tattoo. Her darkening nipples will plump up as the ducts prepare for lactation.

I tell Lila it's too early to listen for her baby's heartbeat, but once she's about twelve weeks we'll listen to it at every visit.

I prepare her for the pelvic exam.

"Do I have to do this *again*? I hate this." She screws up her face and pouts.

I use the smallest speculum. This time, she doesn't clamp her legs shut but sighs loudly, resigned. "I'm only doing this for the baby," she tells me.

In no time, we're done.

"Not too bad, right?"

Lila pushes back and sits up as if she's ready to bolt. But we have some unfinished business.

"So, Lila. You have a black eye. What happened?"

There. Now that everything else is more or less taken care of and Lila is relaxed, I can get around to this. For Lila, it might be the central issue.

She makes a face, kicks her feet. "Freezer door."

"Freezer door?"

"Yeah, my roommate never defrosted it, and it wouldn't shut. I tried to bang it shut but it popped open, hit me right"—she turns and points to her eye, the red patch on her cheek—"here."

The little voice inside me says, *Sure, tell me another one,* yet I had a freezer like that once. After I was divorced from my college-boyfriend husband, I lived alone with our four-year-old daughter and two-year-old son. Their father had taken the car, the camera, and half the wedding gifts and moved west. I had a part-time evening job as a nurse's aide in the local hospital where my son had been born. In the beginning, I had no way to get to work, no money for a down payment on a car, and not enough money for rent, so I advertised for a roommate. She and I shared one bedroom while my kids made room for her son in theirs. We both applied for welfare, and we both enrolled in nursing school. A friend of mine cosigned a loan, and I bought an old gray VW beetle with lots of personality but no backseat.

A few weeks later my application was accepted, and I became, like Lila, a young woman on welfare, a single mom living on the edge. I got a check for half my rent, a coupon book of food stamps, and about one third of what it cost to send my kids to a baby-sitter while I was in nursing school. I signed an agreement promising that after graduation I would work full-time for five years in a local nonprofit hospital. If I didn't, the paper said, I'd have to pay back whatever the state had given me. The system wouldn't help me hunt down the children's father for child support, however. He lived far away, and I didn't have the money to hire an out-of-state lawyer.

I remember two things from that time. One was the damn freezer. It seemed to swell up with ice overnight, and it took hours of thawing and hacking with a screwdriver to get the door closed. The other was the drive-through bank tellers. When my roommate and I handed them our welfare checks, the tellers looked right through us. "No lollipops today," we'd tell the children, who stood on the VW's back floor where the seat should have been, three little towheads steadying themselves, hanging on.

I look again at Lila's fading bruise, her healing temple.

"Is Charles or anyone else giving you trouble these days?"

She stares ahead, arrow straight, as if she were deaf. Lila, tuned out. I know that patients can absorb only so much at one time under the best of circumstances. But when I come too close to the source of their pain, they turn their heads away as if they have caught themselves in the wrong house. Their backs stiffen, and the tension between speaking and silence becomes like static, spark-

ing the air. Sometimes I push, repeat my question, until they release their tears and we can talk about what might help. Not today.

"When did you say you want me back?" Lila asks.

"Two weeks. And here's the number for the women's shelter
hot line. Just in case." I write it on a piece of paper, and she stuffs
it into her jeans. I've learned not to write anything but the number.
That way, when a boyfriend finds the paper and says, "What's
this?" a woman can say whatever she wants. Lila might tell Charles
the truth: "The nurse at the clinic gave it to me. I got to call her if I
have problems."

Her feet tap, and she twists her red hair, now dark blond at the
roots, around her index finger. She's a few pounds heavier than she
was at her last visit, and I think she looks, in spite of her eye, more
rested. Sometimes I can help change a patient's destiny. More often,
it's in her hands.

I hope Lila has a healthy baby. I hope she eats well and drinks
enough milk and doesn't get so depressed that she does drugs or
takes an overdose. I hope her boyfriend stays the hell away from
her. I hope she doesn't pick a fight with her new roommate and
end up on the street. I hope she will call us if she needs anything.
I hope she doesn't disappear from the face of the earth.

"Don't forget to take your vitamins," I offer, unable to find the
words that might help Lila take hold of her life.

Chapter 7

I'm in the middle of an exam in room 6 when I hear loud voices and shouting in the hall. My patient raises her head from the table and looks at me. The voices get louder, and foreboding sounds come to us through the closed door, a muffled thud followed by women's voices, high and piercing, then a prickly silence. The mood of the clinic changes in an instant, as if it were a physical being reacting to some unknown threat, and my own mood changes with it. First there is a hint of unrest, like what a child feels when she's in her bedroom and hears her parents arguing downstairs in hushed tones, only the anger rising up. Then a heavy tension slithers in, like a premonition.

One of the nurses bangs on the exam room door.

"Code Blue," Beth says. "Keep your patient in the room."

"Wait here," I say to the woman lying on the table, and I slip out the cracked-open door. At the end of the corridor across from our secretary's desk, two women are fighting, rolling on the floor and kicking. Their individual arms and legs are indistinguishable, as if they were two figures painted on a twirling ball. The operator's voice twangs over the loudspeaker. "Code Blue, Women's Clinic," it says. "Code Blue, Women's Clinic."

Kate, our secretary, stands over the women, yelling at them

to stop, and the financial counselor, who has ventured out of her office, tries to grab one of them, but the women roll into an even tighter sphere. Then one of them spins free, shattering the whirling circle. She leaps up and runs out our door into the lobby. The other woman chases after her, and I realize that both women are pregnant, five or six months along. They disappear, then wheel and run back into the clinic.

As they sprint toward me, everything seems to move in slow motion. I try to walk, but my arms and legs feel large and weighty, as if I were underwater. Kate's face turns toward me, contorted, and she shouts, "Stay there." Four security guards burst into the clinic, their heavy bodies and buzz-cut heads wagging after the two women, who stop running and begin to punch each other in the belly. The taller woman reaches one hand into her pocket. I curl over, half expecting her to pull out a gun, and one of the security guards propels himself at her like a baseball player lunging for home plate. The tall woman aims a small silver canister right at the other woman's face, and a fog of pepper spray explodes into the air. I turn and cover my face. The sprayed woman's arms jerk up in surprise. She drops to her knees, coughing and gagging.

The guards have caught hold of the taller woman. Their arms surround her middle as she flails at them. Eric, our lone male resident, appears from exam room 4. "Hey, take it easy," he says to the guard. "She's pregnant." Now everyone is choking—the nurses in the hallway, the patients in the waiting room, the security guards who clutch the tall, still-shouting woman. My lungs feel as if I'd inhaled ginger ale.

A policeman arrives, as do three hospital administrators who wear pinstripe suits and cover their faces with handkerchiefs. The sprayed woman is breathless. Water pours from her eyes and nose, and saliva runs from her mouth in ropy strands. I wonder what argument could possibly be worth the risk to their unborn babies? What victory could be worth the potential harm?

"We have to get this one to the ER," says Nina, one of the chief residents, who materializes guiding an empty wheelchair. "And that one," she gestures to the tall woman and back at me, "you examine her before they take her away."

The tall woman and I look at each other.

"Hi, Renée," I say.

She laughs. "Ha. Hi yourself."

———————————

Every once in a while I come across a patient I really don't like. It doesn't happen often, and of course I try not to let the patient know how I feel, but sometimes, in spite of my best efforts, I reveal myself. You'd think a heroin addict would be too out of it to notice, but Renée Jones knows I don't like her. It must be something in the flat tone of my voice, or maybe the way I've tried too hard to be nice. She's had me pegged for years.

She smiles at me. Her teeth are in horrible shape, broken and rotting at the gum line. Her coarse hair is thin and bleached the color of dead straw, her skin pocked with acne. She has a gold stud in one nostril and a gold hoop piercing her left eyebrow. Jail-blue tattoos crawl up and down her coffee-with-cream arms, and her fingernails are bitten down to the quick. Somewhere in there, I always tell myself, is a woman with her own history and funny family stories, someone who dreams and gets up and has good days and bad days, just as I do. I'm just not sure how to find her.

I smile back, my mouth so rigid it might as well be carved in cement. "Come with me," I say, and lead her into an exam room.

"I'm pregnant," she says and smacks her hands on her knees. "Man, I've been trying."

"Your boyfriend's baby?" I remember him: skinny and two feet shorter than Renée.

"Naw, not him. New guy. Really a great guy." She nods her head up and down, up and down.

The first time I met Renée, she was crazy and stoned and had a belly just like this one. That was when I first came to work in the clinic, when I thought I'd already seen it all. In no time, she had me wrapped around her finger.

Every time I saw Renée, she'd grieve over her previous pregnancies, two that had ended in miscarriage and three with scrawny babies the state had taken away. She'd cry and I'd *tsk-tsk* and comfort her. When I measured her belly and asked if she was clean, she'd beam and tell me how, this time, she was *absolutely* staying away from the heroin. "Thanks to you," she'd add.

I'd grin back, full of myself. I'd show the nurses and the residents. I'd keep Renée on the straight and narrow when they had failed.

Time, lots of it, was one of the many things Renée required of me. While I slumped against the wall or sat motionless on my rolling stool, Renée would blubber out the long list of guilty recriminations she kept locked up in her soul. How she'd let her parents down. How she'd ruined the lives of her children. How she'd slept with men when she needed money or sold drugs to kids—oh, she said, that was bad, the worst of all. But no more, she swore to me. Everything was clear to her, the error of her ways and the path back to righteousness.

"No, really, I promise," she'd say. "I *know* I did wrong before, but now I'm smart! I haven't done any stuff in a couple days, yeah, a couple days, and I know I can kick 'cause of this baby here. All the other babies ... well, I don't know where *they* are, but this one's right here." Renée would tap her tight belly, and tears would zigzag down her cheeks.

I realized that her remorse was real, in spite of the residents who warned me that she was just putting on a show to keep me from calling Family Services or spilling tears to keep me sitting by her side. It was then that I adopted a principle I've followed ever since: I decided I would believe that every patient's pain, physical or emotional, was genuine. I would take all patients, especially Renée, at face value. I would believe what they chose to tell me. Even if what they said was not factually true, I knew there was, nevertheless, an emotional truth that I could accept. I learned to listen to the feeling behind the voice, the story behind the words. Trying to second-guess patients was exhausting and disingenuous. Besides, how could patients trust me if I didn't trust them? Surely, I told myself, any woman who had suffered as profoundly as Renée could find the strength to turn her life around.

Renée became my special patient. My project.

"So, Renée," I say. "What was that fight about?"

"Ha, you know, nothing you want to hear. That bitch owes me."

"How pregnant are you?"

"Who knows?"

"Is the baby moving?"

"Yeah, too much."

"Are you having any cramping now?"

Renée doesn't answer. She swipes her hand over her nose. She's lanky as a basketball player, as skittish and haunted as a greyhound. But she sits still and lets me clean the scratches on her face and dab peroxide on the raw patches where hunks of hair have been torn away from her scalp. She's not bleeding vaginally, and the fetal heart tones are strong, but I tell the policeman waiting outside that I still want one of the residents to do a quick ultrasound. Eric comes in, turns off the lights, and scans Renée's belly. In the glow cast by the ultrasound monitor, I make out a maze of needle tracks on Renée's arms, little groundhog burrows at the crook of her elbow. Some of them are old. Others, red punctures in her dilated veins, are new. Her abdomen is scarred, too, skin pops here and there that have healed puckery and maroon.

Eric says, "It's a boy, twenty-one and a half weeks." The baby's heart pumps away on the screen, like a firefly trapped in a jelly jar.

When we're finished, the cop unlocks the handcuff that secured one of Renée's wrists to the side of the exam table. Before he takes her away, Renée winks at me. She knows they won't lock up a pregnant woman for long.

"Renée, please make an appointment to see us," I say. "You need prenatal care."

"Honey, I need more than that." She laughs as the cop hauls her brusquely toward the door.

The last time Renée was pregnant, her baby was stillborn at thirty-seven weeks. "Overwhelming infection," the pathology report said. "Placental abruption." And the mandatory drug screen done after

Renée's delivery was positive for heroin, cocaine, alcohol, and bar-biturates. It was a wonder, they said, that she hadn't died too. So much for my special influence. When I heard, my cheeks burned but I didn't say anything. I was chagrined, humiliated. Didn't she tell me she was clean? Hadn't she had a few negative drug screens during the pregnancy to substantiate her claim? I had been fooled so easily. How could I continue to see patients and believe the emo-tional truth of their words without becoming cynical, hardened to their stories and especially to their tears? I left the baby gift I'd bought for Renée in my locker and went upstairs to visit.

"I really thought you'd make it," I said.

She laughed. "Then you're a bigger fool than me."

Chapter 8

Eleanor's Pap test result had returned three weeks after her initial visit; one of the residents had flagged the report and left it in my box. I'd been surprised when I read the pathologist's notation: "ASCUS," he'd written. "Atypical Squamous Cells of Undetermined Significance. Please repeat."

The pathologist could see that the cervical cells were abnormal, but it wasn't clear why. ASCUS Paps are often caused by inflammation or some other process that temporarily distorts the cervical cells—a yeast infection, a few blood cells left over from a recent menstruation, or even the changes in vaginal discharge that accompany a pregnancy. Sometimes, an ASCUS Pap is an early indication of a more serious condition. Following our standard procedure, I'd called Eleanor and asked her to come back for a second Pap test. She'd remembered me as soon as I said, "Hi. It's Cortney from the women's clinic."

I had reassured her that the next Pap might be fine. I'd also reminded her that she had agreed to return for an endometrial biopsy. "Maybe we could do both tests at the same visit," I'd suggested, but she had shushed me. "Listen," she'd said. "I barely have time to go grocery shopping, let alone spend all my time at the clinic. Anyway, I'm sure there's no reason for concern."

Then, a few weeks ago, she hurried in for her repeat Pap test.

Afterward, rushing out the door, she called back to me. "If this Pap is abnormal," she said, "or if I have any more unusual bleeding, *then* we'll talk about further testing."

Now, Eleanor's chart is back in my message box, her repeat Pap test result clipped to the front. Nina has written across the paper in red ink: "She needs a colpo stat. Do you want to call her?"

OK, I think to myself. So it looks as if Eleanor really does have something going on. Maybe it won't turn out to be a big deal. I'll call her today and get her on the books for a colposcopy, a procedure that allows a resident to take a closer look at the cervix and do some directed biopsies of any suspicious areas. Happens all the time. There are many reasons for an abnormal Pap, and there are many gradations of abnormal.

It's probably that pesky wart virus. Or maybe the cells still look funny because Eleanor's cervix bled once again when I did the second Pap. Sometimes a spot of blood is enough to make a Pap a bit off.

I take the lab report back to the residents' room, and when I read the tiny black computer-printed diagnosis—"Severe dysplasia, marked inflammation, can't rule out adenocarcinoma"—all my easy explanations fly away.

I try to recall what Eleanor's cervix looked like. Had I seen any ulcerated areas? Had I felt any hard nodules or thickenings? I'd placed cervical cancer last on my list of possible reasons for Eleanor's vaginal spotting—she wasn't the typical high-risk patient. She didn't smoke, and she'd had only two sexual partners. But she had contracted human papillomavirus, or HPV, the wart virus, from her first husband, and she hadn't had a Pap test in five years. If she had come in for an exam last year, three years ago, five years ago—would the Pap have been abnormal then? Had her cervical cells been changing and dividing, undetected, all this time?

I call and catch Eleanor at home.

———

"Eleanor?" I say when her voice answers, a "Hello" that isn't tilted up at the end like a question, like most people's hello, but raised in front, "*Hel-*lo," as if I have interrupted her in the midst of great enjoyment.

She tells me she's getting ready to leave to teach her afternoon class, Advanced Geometry. I say that I remember drawing circles and rhomboids that rolled across the page like well-ordered planets. Eleanor doesn't dash ahead, guessing why I've called or letting her imagination run away with her. Instead she allows everything to unfold, as if all things had their own time and place, as if all news came when it was due.

She gives only the slightest intake of breath when I say "another abnormal Pap," and her voice hardly snags when she asks me what happens during the colpo.

"When the resident does the colposcopy, you will be in stirrups as in a regular exam. The resident will put a solution on your cervix to highlight any atypical areas. The colposcope is like a big microscope. The resident looks through it and sees your cervix, magnified. She'll take biopsies of any areas on your cervix that look suspicious, and those samples will go to pathology to be evaluated. Whatever the results, the residents and attending physicians will have a meeting to discuss them and recommend the best treatment. We'll give you an appointment a week after the colpo to talk about what comes next."

I don't tell her that we call this weekly meeting a "Tumor Board" or that the doctors who attend are cancer specialists, radiation oncologists who decide when and how to use the powerful invisible beams that shrink abnormal growths and medical oncologists who measure and prescribe the colorful poisons with lovely names like "cisplatin" and "vincristine," toxic cocktails that fry the cancer cells and in the process damage normal cells as well. Sometimes a woman's hair comes out like clumps of yarn from the head of an old Raggedy Ann doll. Sometimes a woman fights nausea or diarrhea, reassuring herself all the while that these side effects mean that the medicine is, after all, good; that it's doing its arduous work.

"What kind of treatment might they suggest?" Eleanor asks.

I'm evasive: "It depends on the biopsy results. The Pap test is only a screening tool. We need tissue samples to make a diagnosis for sure."

How much do you tell? With how much hope do you balance your bad news?

Long ago, when I was head nurse on an oncology unit, a patient died unexpectedly. I walked into her room, and there she was, mottled and already gone, her belly, once rotund from the swollen liver beneath, now sunk into her bones. I phoned her sisters. First I told them she'd taken a turn for the worse. "Get ready to come in," I said. Then I called back, minutes later, to tell them the situation was grave, that I had called her doctor. The three sisters had time to catch their individual breaths, savor their individual memories. They waited beside the phone for my directive. On the third call, only ten minutes after the first, I told them to come in to the hospital, quickly. I met them at the elevator, and we all rushed in to the cooling body, I and the three sisters with their sturdy cordovan shoes and prepared hearts. I did what I did instinctively, not pausing to wonder if my ruse was ethical. Later the sisters thanked me for not surprising them right off. We'd been playing an ancient game, and they'd been in on it all along.

When Eleanor had been in the office with me, I'd found it easy to reassure her. Now I feel myself step back, withdrawing. If not detected in time, cervical cancer can be fatal. This year, in the United States, about twelve thousand cases of cervical cancer will be discovered. Almost five thousand women will die.

There is silence on the other end of the line. Eleanor might be slipping on her sweater, wishing I would hurry. How long will her students wait for her? Is she a professor or just an adjunct instructor?

"So is this a serious problem?" she asks me in her teacher's voice.

"It could be," I reply, searching for the words to change doctor talk into people talk. "Abnormal Paps can be caused by many things, inflammation or minor infections as well as cancer. But cervical cancer, discovered in time, can be curable."

If I stay positive, if I can transmit positive energy, maybe

Eleanor's cervical cells will straighten themselves out, line up like inexperienced recruits who have fallen out of formation. After all my time in health care, I still believe in magic. I do know that the body is a miraculous thing. I also believe the spirit can sometimes change fate.

"Oh" is all she says. Most women greet the news of a second abnormal Pap with a zillion questions that reveal the content of their fears.

I close out the noise around me, ignore a child's laughter coming in from some exam room. I feel the walls around me come to attention. But all she asks is "How soon can I have this colposcopy done?"

"I've made an appointment for you already," I say. "Next Friday at nine-thirty in the morning."

I find myself buoyed by her businesslike manner, by the strength I feel growing within her. I decide to accept this image: Eleanor as a resister.

"Do you have any questions for me?" I ask. Not that I have any of the answers. Even the pathologist—master of cellular nuance, of the strange encryption of disease—doesn't yet have an answer.

"No," she says. "Not now. If I do I'll call you back." Eleanor, in a rush to be off to school.

"Thank you," she adds. "I'm sure everything will be fine."

Although it is my job to comfort her, Eleanor has reassured me. I wonder if she believes in magic, too, or if she's simply fighting to maintain control. I wonder if she will weep or call a friend after we hang up. Or if, in order to keep the reality of her abnormal Pap test at bay, she will simply go teach her class, hiding any sign of distress from her young and healthy students, just as I sometimes hide my emotions, leaving one patient and entering the next patient's room with a smile.

As I do now. I say good-bye to Eleanor and pick up the next patient's chart, walk in, and greet her as if she's the only one on my mind. As if I'd never found a lump in anyone's breast, or found a pregnancy that would inevitably miscarry, or given anyone bad news.

Chapter 9

"The pain is no better," Joanna says. "In fact, it's even worse."

She couldn't wait for her follow-up appointment but called asking if she could come back to my evening clinic *sooner.* When I reviewed Joanna's chart and read my last note, I realized how much I had left out of that official record, how much we caregivers always leave out. All my intuitive worries, everything I'd thought about Joanna as I drove home after our first appointment, my concerns about the disparity between her smile and her anxiety and my debate with myself whether to mention this to her or not— none of that appears in my note. Instead, my summation is brief: "32 year old woman who has never been pregnant, currently in a long-term relationship using birth control pills, here tonight complaining of three-month history of pelvic pain and vaginal burning that occurs only with intercourse."

"Even worse," I say, a statement more than a question, and sit down. I've barely gotten in the door. I wanted to greet Joanna and say hello, but instead I find myself propelled right into the medical mode.

I pull up my stool so we are face to face, almost knee to knee, a friendly approach. Then I roll back, just the slightest bit, to a clinical distance.

"It's really bad," she says, combing her hair with her fingers.

She is wearing a long indigo skirt that flares out at the bottom, a matching tunic top, black sandals with short rolled socks, and strands of multicolored beads that jiggle around her neck, giving her an artistic, festive look, as if she might be on her way to a painting exhibit or a dance. Her face, however, is immobile and pallid. Tonight, Joanna is not smiling.

"I kept a record," she says, and hands me a small tan pocket calendar, the pages neatly rubber-banded to the present week. I undo the band and look back over the days. She has marked the eight times in the past weeks that she and David had sex. On each of these days, she has written "Pain!" in red ink in large, loopy handwriting. Sometimes the day after has a red "Pain!" as well. The other days are blank.

"I'm sorry, Joanna. The lubricant didn't seem to make any difference," I say, handing the book back to her.

"I tried putting it on me and then putting it on him, but it didn't help. Maybe just in the beginning, then it seemed to disappear and I still got irritated."

Joanna looks at me. Her cheeks are burnished. I wonder, when she gets irritated during sex, if she gets emotionally irritated as well. At David or at herself. She's waiting for me, I know, to make some pronouncement. Usually I'm good at bringing order into out-of-control places, soothing a woman into an exam or making the difficult exam easier, forewarning of pain and how to control it. But this encounter seems off already. I feel harried, out of step.

"Your chlamydia and gonorrhea cultures came back negative," I say.

"Then why am I still having pain? And this swelling. There must be something else going on."

"Pelvic pain can have many causes. And sometimes the problem might not be related to your uterus or ovaries, but to other organs. Your intestines, your bladder. Sometimes it takes awhile to figure it out."

"So what am I supposed to do? I'm beginning to think I'm crazy or something. Last night it hurt so much, he stopped."

"He stopped?"

Joanna looks across the room. "Well, if David sees that it hurts, he stops."

"What if he doesn't notice? Do you tell him?"

She looks back. "Usually not," she says. What I hear is *I tolerate it. I'm afraid to say anything.*

The small voice inside me, the one that is never recorded in the official documents, prods me to ask, "Why don't you tell him?" and all my senses are signaling as well, urging me to take action. I *do* see Joanna's flat expression, I hear the submission in her voice, my hands want to reach over and take hers. But Joanna has turned away again, and there's something about her prickly defense, her desperately controlled anxiety, that silences me. I'm afraid if I say the wrong thing, Joanna will shatter into pieces.

"Have you tried any medication that helps? Advil or Tylenol?" I ask. I'm ashamed of myself for letting that moment pass, but still, I don't go back to it.

"Well, I can't take anything because I never know when it's going to happen. I can't take pills all the time, can I?"

I shake my head no. I have my arms locked around my knee, and I'm sitting in what must look like a casual position, tilted slightly back on my rolling stool, contemplating Joanna as she speaks. But I feel as though I'm up against a barricade. She's angry with me. I haven't been able to snap my fingers and erase her pain. I'm upset with myself, too. There's a missing clue, and, although I have an idea what it might be, I can't seem to shake it loose. So far, wherever I search for a handhold, a chink to hook my fingers through, I find solid rock.

"Joanna, has the nature of the pain changed at all in the past few weeks? Other than getting worse?"

"It happens all the time. When he first enters me, then when he moves. Now it hurts for two days after he's finished." She articulates this difficult information mechanically, as if she were reading a script or talking about someone else.

"After he's finished," I repeat.

"Yes, you know, after we have sex." When she looks down, her hair swings across her cheek, a sharp angle.

"Have you and David talked about this?" I wonder if they've tried increasing the amount of foreplay or maybe talked about not having sex at all for a while.

"I told him I think I have a problem. He's worried too. He said he'll do anything to help me. He suggested maybe we should see someone together."

"That would be a good idea," I say. "I can suggest some wonderful counselors." There is no response from Joanna, so I shift direction. "Tell me more about David."

Joanna feels the change. She crosses her legs.

"I left New York six months ago to move in with him. We've been together five or six years. I don't know how he puts up with this." Joanna clicks her nails against her rings, silver bands she wears on her right hand. "David is really a great guy."

"Did you have this pain with any other partners? Or with David before the last few months?"

"No," she says. "It only started recently."

"Can you think of anything that might have triggered this pain? For example, has anything changed in your relationship? Anything different since you moved in with him?"

I keep waiting for her to give me information willingly and all in a jumble, as many women do. They open their treasure chest of facts and tumble them out for me to sort through. If there is anything, Joanna's keeping it to herself.

"No, nothing," she says. "Not that I can think of."

For a few moments, neither of us speaks. Usually such a lapse doesn't bother me, but with Joanna there seems to be an urgency about the silence, a void that I find myself pressured to fill. This is crazy, I say to myself. She's the patient, and *I'm* the one who's hyperalert, my whole body ready to duck some unseen blow. Maybe, I think, I should pay attention to this. Perhaps I'm expressing what she can't.

I've already asked her, but I ask again: "Joanna, are you being physically or emotionally abused in any way? By David or by anyone else? It's so common that I always ask all my patients."

"You asked me before," she says.

"Yes, I did."

"No," she says. "David is wonderful to me. If anything, I've never felt so safe."

"Sometimes," I say, "issues come up when we feel safe enough to address them."

Joanna turns her head. She hunches her shoulders and tucks her hands under her thighs again, as if by doing so she could shelter her body and protect all the vulnerable soft parts.

OK, I think, *try something else.* Once I watched a sailboat race, a whole regatta of polished, swift beauties. When a wind came up, threatening to take them off course, the sailors scrambled to swing their sails about, tacking into the wind. The sails chattered and deflated, then suddenly they cracked open, the air tightening each sail into an arc. The boats sped off, headed for the finish line. I wonder if I can catch anything by tacking about, scooping up any information that will help Joanna and me find our way.

"Joanna, did you tell me where your family lives?"

"Ohio," she says. She has one younger brother and one older sister, both living with their spouses near her father in Cleveland. She's the only sibling still not married. Her mother died several years ago in a car accident. Joanna moved to New York after college, determined to live a different life.

"So you're the rebel," I say. "The one who got away. How does your family feel about that?"

"They weren't happy. The first time I left Ohio, I went to Italy to study art for two years. Then I moved to New York. And I haven't told them I moved in with David. 'Get married and have some kids and give up this idea about being an artist,' my dad says."

I nod. "Are you going to tell him you moved in with David?"

"I don't know," she says.

"Worrying about your family's reaction could certainly increase your stress level," I say.

"Do you think this is all in my mind?" she snaps, surprising me. So there is a wildfire raging in Joanna. One finger of flame just leapt out.

"Not at all," I say. "I'm just trying to figure out what might be different for you since you began having this problem."

Instantly, she's composed again. "The only thing I'm stressed about, I suppose, is my business. It's hard for me to get new clients this far from the city. I keep running back and forth."

"Sometimes stress can affect sexuality. If you're under a lot of pressure, making love to David may be just one more demand."

Joanna doesn't answer. "There must be something else you can do," she says.

"There is. I think we should get an ultrasound to take a better look."

"What will that show?" she says.

"It may show a cyst or fibroid that's too small for me to feel but enough to cause pain. When you have intercourse, your partner's penis contacts your cervix, moving it and jostling your uterus and ovaries as well. If there's a small ovarian cyst, if there's a uterine anomaly—any of these things can increase the pain."

"What if the ultrasound is OK?"

"Depending on what the ultrasound shows and depending on what happens with the pain, I may ask you to see a medical doctor, too, to make sure there's nothing else going on. I think it would be helpful for you and David to see a counselor as well."

Joanna's psyche is quick and agile. It sidesteps completely my inference that there may be an emotional component to this pelvic pain.

"But what happens if the medical doctor finds there *is* nothing else wrong. Then what?"

"Then," I say, "I'd consider referring you to the chief residents for further evaluation. But I don't think that's where this is headed. Why not get the ultrasound first, and then we'll take it from there?"

"I don't want you to examine me tonight," she says.

"That's fine, Joanna." Actually, I'm happy that she's declining an exam. Maybe that means she's beginning to trust me enough to refuse.

"How soon can I have the ultrasound?"

I take out a prescription pad and write, "Abdominal and trans-vaginal pelvic ultrasound, diagnosis: pelvic pain for three months," sign my name, and give the slip to Joanna. "The department is closed in the evening," I say, "but I'll call you tomorrow with a date and time."

There's a part of me that doesn't feel adequate to the task of solving the enigma of Joanna's pain, and this realization leaves me both sad and somewhat relieved. I want to be able to see Joanna through this. If I can't, I can always refer her on to one of the chief residents or to one of our attending gynecologists. Joanna wants me to find some visible, explainable reason for her symptoms, and she wants me to make that physical *thing* go away. I think we're chasing after something much less tangible, a series of events, perhaps, or maybe only a moment. I'm convinced that the cause of Joanna's pelvic pain has more to do with a bruise in her soul than with an abnormality in her body. But I'm not ready to give up yet.

I imagine Joanna as a young student, leaving Ohio to stroll the museums in Rome and Florence. I wonder if, like me, she admired the work of Giotto, how he created the illusion of depth on a flat, frescoed wall, and how he drew a faint outline around his madonnas and saints, both illuminating and restraining them. From the little I have seen, it appears that Joanna must also live in two worlds: one where her artistic imagination is unfettered and free; the other where something dangerous and deeply repressed must be kept under tight control.

Chapter 10

Usually I go for a mammogram every year, faithfully, just as I urged Eleanor to do. March for mammogram, I figure, a good way to remember. But this year I kept putting it off. March came and went. I decided to wait until after my vacation. After all, my mammograms had always been negative. I waited until after my granddaughter's April birthday, then until after our driveway was paved, as if every event were a rational excuse. June was just around the corner when I finally called for an appointment.

The whole process was over in no time and seemed mostly like an inconvenience. I had to dash up from the clinic in between patients, disrobe, wait for the tech to develop the films, then go back to the clinic with my breasts still tingling, two throbbing red lines etched on my skin where the Plexiglas plates had slid down the slope of my chest and compressed the tissue. Within an hour, all these discomforts were gone. Two days later, I received a letter that said I had to return for further testing, "special compressions of one specific area." There was something in there; something the radiologist had seen.

As dutifully as any patient, I returned to the small room and the large green machine on the third floor. I waited with the other women lined up on the brown plastic sofa, all of us in shabby white gowns, all of us nervously scanning magazines, pretending to be fascinated by recipes or articles on spring bulbs. I was the third woman in line. Finally, the tech called me in, told me to drop my gown. She studied my original mammogram on the view box, then used a small round disk to compress the breast once again, aiming at that one particular renegade spot.

After I dressed, the radiologist beckoned me into his back room. He knew I was a nurse practitioner. Would he tell me what he'd tell any patient, or would he give me more details, expecting me to be clinical, objective? In the dark, I sat perched on a high stool next to him, the new mammogram at eye level, black and white and magnified. He pointed to the image of my right breast.

"See here?" He squinted, wrinkling his nose as if that would help him focus. "Just beneath the curve of the areola? Micro-calcifications, more than ten of them, in a cluster." I saw them, too, chalk white against the graphite gray of the normal tissue: white squiggles like tiny worms, freeze-framed and suspended in time.

The radiologist leaned in to study the microcalcifications, then directed my attention to a chart hung on the wall beside the view box. In the dim light, I strained to make it out.

"See the top two lines? Those are pictures of benign micro-calcifications. When we see these, we usually repeat the mammo in six months." I didn't see *my* microcalcifications there. Mine were different. Smaller, more linear, like long grains of rice that had accidentally been spilled in one small area on the film, or like radioactive dust.

"And, looking back," he said, pulling down this mammogram and clipping last year's in its place, "I notice that there were some early changes then, but they were almost impossible to see." He traced the area for me. Even so, I could barely distinguish them, a few ghostly shadows nestled deep in the tissue.

"Now that we know where they are, we can see them. So the microcalcifications have been there more than a year, and they're increasing." He snapped off the view box and flipped on the room light. My eyes watered, and I blinked like someone coming out of a movie theater at midday.

"What do you recommend?" I asked.

"If you were my wife," he said, "I'd want the area biopsied."

"If you were my wife," the gold standard of medical care, something patients ask all the time—*What would you do if it were you, Doc, or someone in your family*—but doctors, unwilling to influence a patient incorrectly, usually reserve this kind of privileged advice for someone in the fold—another doctor, a nurse practitioner. I nodded.

"Yes," I said.

Suddenly breast cancer had become a neighbor, not a stranger from another town. She had moved in next door to me, and she was walking up my front steps. I wondered what she wanted. A cup of flour? Or something more? To take over my family, wear my clothes, and lie in bed at night with my husband?

Usually, doctors and nurses gain authority not only by their titles but also by the expectations patients hold of them. Patients think we're in charge, the privileged ones with the sacrosanct information. But when caregivers become patients, we, too, are reduced to the essence of our bodies: the bitten nails, the stretch marks, the festering blemish. I felt myself shedding my white coat and forgetting how to use my stethoscope. All I wanted was a doctor who would know what was wrong and which treatment would cure me, and nurses who would keep me safe and free from pain. Like any other patient, I wanted to go through the bad time, the sick time, and emerge unscathed.

"Certainly," I agreed. "Of course I want it biopsied."

I stared straight ahead into the shiny glass of the view box and saw myself staring back. The radiologist leaned his hands on the counter in front of us and turned away from my reflection to look at me.

"As you know, microcalcifications are just small fragments of calcium that show up on the mammogram. They could represent a number of things. Seventy-five percent of the time, they're nothing, benign calcium in an aging vessel or an old degenerating fibroadenoma."

I nodded again, thinking about the 25 percent remaining, the precancerous 25 percent. Even though I knew the statistics—that it can take years for precancerous microcalcifications to evolve into a palpable cancerous mass—I didn't feel reassured. I felt as if something foreign had been in my breast all along and I hadn't even known. Now that I knew, my body suddenly seemed different. Now I understood what my patients meant when they found out they had an infection, or a cyst on their ovaries, or an abnormal test and said they felt *invaded.*

I thanked the doctor, telling him I would call my surgeon for an appointment. Then I returned to the clinic to finish my shift. For the rest of the day, I felt a kinship with my patients that went beyond the usual. Now I was one of them. I was especially careful to explain everything fully, to pause and ask again, "Do you have any questions?"

I spent the days before the breast biopsy planning how I would cope if the diagnosis were cancer. I wanted to be an example to my children, my husband, and my patients. Somehow, I imagined, I would be made transcendent and special by my illness. Other women with cancer would welcome me as the newest member of a dread society. We would know what no one else could, and we would recognize one another on the street by the stunned look in our eyes. I would see everything differently, I thought, cherishing each day and not wasting a moment. That's what I pretended. Inside, I was paralyzed.

Everyone I told about my impending biopsy had a story to relate—about women they knew who'd had breast cancer, which ones had narrowly escaped. A close friend told me that she'd recently heard from three college pals. Each of them had breast cancer. "It's like an epidemic," she said. My friend figured it was only a matter of time until she developed breast cancer, too, just as her mother and her friends had. "But I don't feel hopeless," she said. "Every time I hear about someone else who recovers, I know that it's possible."

Two nurses who'd had breast cancer, per diem employees who work in the clinic when the regular nurses are sick or on vacation, tried to cheer me up. "Even if it is malignant," they said, "it's so early you have a good chance of cure." They wore their own experiences with breast cancer bravely. I asked them everything—about the biopsy, the surgery, the radiation, the chemotherapy. I wanted to know what it was like for them. *Not knowing* and *not naming* seemed to give breast cancer a power it didn't deserve. I said "malignant" and "chemo" and "tumor" as often as I could, in case those words might soon apply to me. If I knew everything, even the worst, it wouldn't be as bad and I wouldn't be so afraid. At work, when I have to give a difficult diagnosis, I always ask my patients, "Tell me how much you'd like to know." I wanted to know everything.

"What was the chemo like?" I asked Pat, one of the per diem nurses.

"Didn't bother me a bit. I had a wonderful nurse. Every time she gave me my chemo, she'd tell me not to go home and feel sorry for myself. So I went shopping."

First she'd get the injection, then she'd wrap her bald head in a turban and go to the mall. Now when she laughs, she laughs with her whole body, celebrating the smallest kindness, the most minor pleasure. In the clinic, she's the one who supports patients the most, who runs to exclaim over a newborn. I love to watch her move about the world. If I do have cancer, I said to myself, that's how I'll be.

Chapter 11

*My biopsy wasn't scheduled until 11 A.M. When I arrived in the one-*day surgical unit, the nurse told me to get undressed in the small, pleasant cubicle complete with TV, plush carpeting, and private bathroom. With the removal of each item of my clothing—my faded blue T-shirt, my jeans, my tan sandals, my watch, my bra and underpants—I became more and more a patient. The more naked I became, the more difficult it was for me to locate the "I" who was also a mother and a nurse, a writer and a wife.

Ten minutes after I put on the striped robe and paper slippers, a transporter knocked, and then loaded me onto a stretcher and rolled me down to radiology. The first step in a breast biopsy is to localize the area in question—the lump or, in my case, the micro-calcifications. Because these changes can be invisible to the eye, a surgeon has to have some guideline, some road map into the breast, to be able to find the lesions and then excise the correct portion of tissue. About a half hour before the actual biopsy, a mammogram is done to calculate the angle and depth of the mass or calcifications. While the breast is compressed, a radiologist places a needle through the skin and threads a thin wire, called Kopan's wire, through the needle into the target area. No local anesthetic is used. It might swell and distort the tissue, making accurate placement impossible.

So once again I faced the mammography machine, this time perched on a tall stool so I didn't have to stand. "We have to keep your breast under pressure for quite a while," the tech said. "And sometimes that makes women feel faint."

She slipped my gown off. The room was cold.

She asked me to lean forward. Then she picked up my right breast and smoothed it flat on the Plexiglas plate, adjusting it as if it were a piece of wrinkled linen she was about to iron. The bulk of my breast felt strange, detached from me. Another tech changed the top plate. The new plate had several holes in it.

"We'll take a picture, then the doctor will insert the needle through one of these openings," the first woman said. "We'll check its placement with another picture. We have to keep you compressed the whole time."

The plates came down, inch by inch, with a grinding sound. My right arm was hooked up and over the frame, my shoulder twisted out of the way. As my breast thinned and flattened under the steady pressure until it grew numb, I looked around the room and chatted with the techs about their jobs and the latest hospital news. I tried to ignore my nudity and my contorted position and my hands that were so cold my fingernails were dusky blue. Denial was the only way I could hold on to any sense of *wellness*.

The techs hid behind the lead shield, and the machine chugged and took the first X ray, a series of gruff coughs. They left the room to develop the film and show it to the radiologist, who would do his calculations and then insert the guide needle into my breast. I waited in the room, corkscrewed on my pedestal. The techs were gone ten minutes. It felt as if they'd left me alone for half an hour.

"Sorry," one of them said, coming in with another whoosh of cold air. "It's a zoo out there. You know how it is. He's right in the middle of another procedure."

In five minutes, the radiologist hurried in. My head was turned so I couldn't see him, but it wasn't the man I'd spoken to before.

"I'm Dr. Gilman," this new voice said. "I'm going to insert the needle now. This usually doesn't bother women too much."

I assumed that meant I wasn't supposed to feel any pain, or at least not to *say* that I did. I found myself wanting to live up to his expectations.

He twirled the stylus through one of the holes on the top plate. A sharp heat pierced the core of my breast. I felt a bit light-headed. "There, that wasn't too bad," he said and hastened away. The silver marker stuck out of my breast like a flag.

The techs took another picture to make sure the point was in the right place. Again they left. My shoulder, still twisted around, ached. When I felt faint, I took deep, slow breaths.

"OK, you're almost all set," they said, dropping the metal X-ray plates onto the counter as they breezed in. They relieved the pressure on my breast a bit, and we waited for the radiologist to return. We talked some more about our families, about the problems in their department.

"You know," they said. "Same politics in the clinic, right?"

I wished they wouldn't talk about work. I wished they would treat me like a patient and not like a coworker. If I were a patient, I could say that I felt faint, that I was frightened, that the pain in my breast felt like a white-hot burn. As a coworker, I had to be jovial. Complicit and gossipy.

The radiologist came back to remove the outer sheath of the needle, a thick nauseating tugging that left the Kopan's wire in place, the end of it splayed open inside my breast like a tiny arrow pointing the way. During the surgery, my doctor would use his scalpel to follow this wire. At the base of it, right where the end splayed out, lurked the invisible microcalcifications.

The techs taped the flexible wire down to my skin and placed a bulky gauze pad on top. "I don't want to lie down," I said as they helped me back onto the stretcher. Instead I sat up, wanting to see where we were going as the transporter pushed me back to the elevator, up to the fourth floor, and into the surgery suite, where he parked me in a small alcove outside the main operating room desk, sliding me in face out, as if my stretcher were a compact car that he skillfully maneuvered. Next to me a bunch of mops leaned against the wall.

While I waited, I watched the OR secretary. A green cap covered her hair. Her green scrub gown was tied in front with a stingy bow. Every once in a while she looked up at me, but she didn't say anything. I tried to look intelligent and composed, as if I were there simply to observe.

"Your doctor is on his way," said another woman with reddish hair and big beige glasses who appeared from around the corner. "I'm your anesthesiologist, and I'm going to start your IV."

She said her name too fast for me to understand.

"I'm only having local, no conscious sedation," I responded, trying to remember to use the right words, the official ones.

Her eyebrows, the same color beige, arched over the tops of her glasses. "Oh?" she said. "So I'm not going to be needed in the room?"

"I don't think so," I answered.

A nurse came up to the other side of my stretcher. She didn't introduce herself but said, "I spoke to your doctor. He wants you to have an IV anyway, just in case we need to give you something."

My heart started to pound, *poom, poom, poom, poom.* All of a sudden I was losing my grip on the sense of wellness I'd been clutching all along. If I could just manage to hold on to it, if any patient could, then we'd be the equals of the health care team, not their victims or passive recipients. We'd have the power and the authority to say what we could and could not tolerate. They'd hear us tell them what *we* needed to get through *their* procedures.

The anesthesiologist started my IV line and taped it with three slender strips of transparent tape, and the fluid crept into my vein, a cold finger tracing a line up the tender part of my inner arm. The nurse rolled my stretcher into the OR, past the scrub tech who stood guarding her instruments. I slid over onto the table, black and narrow and chilly as snakeskin.

I heard my doctor's voice in the hallway, a deep ribbon of sound. As the nurse tightened the blood pressure cuff around my arm, I heard his footsteps, then, as he bent over me, I saw Dr. Patino's brown eyes over his green mesh mask, my eyes mirrored in his pupils. He'd never operated on me before, but his was the name everyone mentioned. "He's the man if you have a breast lesion," the doctors had told me. Every woman I had spoken to had said the same thing, but they had mentioned his humanity as well as his expertise. "He's wonderful," they had told me. "Caring and gentle."

"It's freezing in here," he said. "It's very important to the success of the operation that you're comfortable." Then he asked for towels, and the nurse brought big white ones fresh from the warmer. He wrapped warm towels around my head and neck, and one around each arm. He clicked the latch on the table and bent my knees, sliding a pillow beneath them. He asked for slippers for my feet, then wrapped another warm towel around my legs. Sometimes nurses are as smart as doctors, just as good at diagnosing what's wrong or knowing what to do. Sometimes doctors are as compassionate and comforting as nurses.

While the nurse washed my breast with foamy soap that trickled into my armpit and under my back, Dr. Patino went to the anteroom to scrub. The nurse slipped a metal plate under my hip, a ground that would allow the surgical team to use the electrocautery, the Bovie, without shocking me. This instrument can be used to cauterize bleeding vessels or to carve through tissue like a knife. Just before the doctor returned to inject my breast with local anesthetic, the nurse drew a heavy green sheet over the frame that arched above my head. The OR suite disappeared, and under the tented sheet everything appeared verdant, watery. My breath was hot, and slowly my face warmed. The numbing medication infiltrated my breast, and I felt the doctor's hands begin to tug and press.

When he used the cautery, small tingles traveled through me from my breast to my back. When the tissues were burned and sealed, the odor of singed flesh rose in the air and seeped through the fibers of my tent. If I closed my eyes, I could separate myself and leave my breast there on the table under my team's capable hands. When the nurse turned on the radio and tuned in an oldies station, I tapped my feet to songs I remembered from the sixties and seventies, and the scrub tech and I hummed along. Every once in a while, the nurse leaned down and whispered in my ear, "Everything is going fine. Are you OK?"

There was one thing, I realized, that joined us there in that room, the doctor, the nurse, the scrub tech, and me. We were all hungry to know the microcosm of the body, to solve its riddles and understand its intricacies. At various times, we had all rejoiced when the body's hidden parts had willingly revealed themselves. There was the tortuous ear canal we could peer into with our little lights, and the body's hallways, vagina and throat and long sinuous vessels we could navigate with shiny steel instruments and flexible catheters. There was elastic muscle and tissue, and the intestines, translucent and the gorgeous color of salmon. And there was the skin, which guarded its contents fiercely yet, when necessary, yielded easily to the knife. I love the body, I thought from deep in my foresty shelter, even when it betrays us. I remembered the many courageous patients I'd known during my years in health care and the many unforgettable moments I'd experienced, moments of horror or astonishing acts of love: holding a man's heart in my hand during surgery; watching residents practice their surgical skills on a corpse; the psychotic woman who ran out of the intensive care unit with a mattress strapped to her back; the burned boy whose polyester pants had melted to his legs; the physician who stood in Labor and Delivery, rocking and singing, cradling a dying premature boy in his arms because the parents were too shocked to do so; the dying man who escaped from the hospital to run naked in the snow for the last time; the father who performed postmortem care on his son; the nun who bled to death, her blood becoming iridescent stars on the ceiling and walls; the man on the ventilator who, when he awakened, told me that he'd heard everything I said to him night after night, that I was the one who had kept him holding on to life.

How fortunate I was to be not at the beginning of my career, as this young nurse was—all the things she didn't yet know and hadn't yet been privileged to see!—but, like Dr. Patino, well along my way. How lucky I would be if I could keep on loving the body's power and its frailties equally, with compassion and tenderness.

"There," the doctor said, and I felt his hands lift up and away from me, pulling a nickel-sized piece of flesh out of the small crater in my breast. An orderly was summoned to rush the biopsy back to radiology, where it would be X-rayed to confirm the presence of all the microcalcifications seen on the original mammogram. We waited in the OR, harmonizing to Simon and Garfunkel's greatest hits.

After the radiologist phoned to say yes, they're all here, the cluster of white calcium like sprinkles of iridescent rice, and after Dr. Patino closed the flap he'd opened in my breast, sewing the curve of my areola with layers of fine suture, I left the OR in a wheelchair, waving good-bye to the silent secretary in the green cap as the nurse whizzed me past. The biopsy went on to Pathology, where it would be studied, and then, in a few days, I would know.

Even now, a faint lavender blotch still overlies the gentle dent left in my right breast by the surgery. Although I'm wiser than I was as a teenager in Dr. Riley's office, this experience confirmed what I already knew but now understood more than ever: it's not easy to be a female patient. Because most of our reproductive organs are internal, even routine examinations and procedures in the field of women's health are uncommonly invasive, reminding us of our vulnerability. To investigate much of the female body, we must dilate, probe, reach deep.

In addition, almost every female organ represents not only the *real* but the *symbolic*—breasts, which serve for both lactation and pleasure; the vagina, which allows birth and yet becomes, both in literature and in jokes, the forbidden passageway; the uterus, which nests our babies yet is named our enemy when no longer needed—and so manipulation of these areas reverberates emotionally as well as physically. All these organs represent both the sensual and the sexual, the grace of procreation as well as the primal urge, the innocence of girlhood and the involution of senescence. A parallel for men might be the penis and, even more, the hidden prostate, a chestnut-sized gland snugged in the pelvic cavity and wrapped around the beginning of a man's urethra. Remove the prostate, sever the nerves, and a man may become impotent.

To have his prostate examined, a man must curl up like a fetus, expose himself, and tolerate once a year, like a woman, an examiner's gloved finger.

––––––––––––––

My biopsy was negative. Dr. Patino called me on a Friday afternoon, one day after the surgery. I thought he was calling simply to check up on me. I never imagined he'd have a diagnosis from Pathology so soon.

"Hello there," he said. "How are you feeling?"

I was happy to hear his voice. I had no expectations. "My breast is tender," I replied, "and there's some bruising." Actually, my breast was sore, throbbing under the ice pack. Alongside my breast there was an ugly purple blotch that extended along my ribs and pooled under my armpit.

"How about swelling?" he asked.

"Not too bad."

"Well," he said. "Great."

Then, almost as an afterthought, he said, "I'm very pleased to tell you that the biopsy is negative."

My first reaction was simply surprise. "You have the diagnosis already?"

"Yes. I asked them to rush it. I'm going to see you in a week to take out the stitches, right?"

"Right," I said. Then, "Thank you. Thank you so much."

After I hung up, I waited to feel a deep sense of relief. I had been spared. I wanted tears to come to my eyes, I wanted to laugh or call up my family and tell them, I wanted to go for a walk and praise every beautiful thing along the way. But instead I stood in the middle of the kitchen and a quiet, eerie calm settled over me, as if a cloud had drifted in front of the sun, stopping the light flowing in through the windows. I had been riding a high crest of tension and uncertainty, holding my breath. Then, just as a wave crashes against the sand and gently disperses, the tension was gone. I *had* been spared, and for that I was wildly grateful. But a lesser sensation, a kind of fearful apprehension, had quickly moved in.

I wondered how my patients felt when I called *them* up with good news. Did they celebrate, or did they also enter this state of suspended anticipation, wondering "What next?" Did they think, because I moved on to other patients' problems, that I had abandoned them or become unavailable to answer their questions, which, like mine, were no doubt vague and difficult to articulate but nonetheless troubling?

I was left, like my patients, with many uncertainties. Because I'd had these microcalcifications, would I develop more? Should I stop the estrogen I'd been taking ever since my hysterectomy, a medication that stimulates the breast tissue and, according to some studies, increases the risk of cancer? If I did continue the estrogen, would I need a mammogram every six months instead of every twelve? And there was that other question, the one I asked myself only in the middle of the night: Was this the beginning of the aging process, that series of small, unannounced alterations to which we all have to adjust?

My questions remained. When I was a child, I believed that doctors knew everything and could cure any illness. All we had to do was place ourselves in their hands. I'd come to learn that the body is not predictable or reliable—anything about it could change in an instant—and that medicine is only a collection of ever-evolving suppositions, volumes of opinions and differing recommendations. And so I tried to practice what I tell my patients: explore the options, listen to the experts, consult with a trusted adviser, and make the best decision with the information now available. Such routine advice takes on added importance for women when we find ourselves searching for answers. As I combed journals for information on the prevention of breast cancer and Eleanor searched the library for ways to make sense of her abnormal Pap test. As Joanna convinced herself that there must be a physical reason for her pelvic pain and Lila asked her friends what it's like to have a baby.

Chapter 12

*Lila ambles right past me, her baggy pants unsnapped, her high-*top sneakers untied. The purple-green rim around her eye is almost invisible now. If you didn't know she'd had a black eye, you'd think she just looked tired.

"Hi there." I reach out and tap her arm.

"Oh, hey," she says, stops a moment. Coyly, she tilts her head and looks at me. "I came for my ultrasound."

She seems excited, like any young mother about to see her baby for the first time. But unlike other mothers, Lila struggles not to look too happy, too eager.

"Good for you," I say. "Be sure and ask for a picture."

"Cool," she says, absentmindedly tugging her hair. Her beat-up backpack hangs off one shoulder, and a bunch of keys dangles on her hip. She has another key around her neck, suspended on what looks like one of those red-green-blue braided plastic lanyards kids make in summer camp.

"So, is Charles here with you?" I lean back against South America, trying to avoid the pins that run from Nicaragua to Brazil, and Lila leans back against the opposite wall, near the phone.

"Guess not," she says.

I wonder how Lila feels about Charles not finding time to

come see his baby, but she gives me no clues. We lean for a few more seconds.

"Why, you wanna come in with me?" she says. "Or you too busy?"

I am busy. I just saw one patient, and there's another chart waiting, but Lila's taking a giant first step. She's asking for company.

"Sure, I'll come in with you, Lila. I'd like to see this little kid."

She shrugs. "Come on, then."

I follow Lila's half-red hair and shabby backpack down the hall, around the bend to the two small rooms with a grand name, Perinatal Testing Center, where we do ultrasounds and amniocenteses as well as nonstress tests, all the different types of monitoring we use to assess an unborn baby's well-being.

Because Lila's a smoker, she'll have several nonstress tests during the last weeks of her pregnancy. A nurse will secure a fetone, a special stethoscope, to Lila's belly with a fleecy strap, and while she reclines in a leather chair, her baby's magnified heartbeat will trace a jagged line on the monitor screen. With every kick or squirm, the baby's heartbeat should quicken, making a tiny spike on the checkered monitor paper. If the heartbeat accelerates normally with movement, we'll say the strip is "reactive," reassuring us that the baby's heart is still receiving adequate oxygen in spite of the placental vessels being narrowed by Lila's smoking.

Because Lila's young and doesn't have any abnormal genetic history, she's not a candidate for an amniocentesis, a test we offer to women over thirty-five and to those at risk of having babies with genetic abnormalities: women with Down syndrome relatives, women who've had a baby with cardiac or other defects, women whose screening blood tests indicate possible problems. First the woman's belly is numbed. Then the resident inserts a long, shiny needle under ultrasound guidance, piercing the skin and the muscle, penetrating the uterine wall, and entering the amniotic space, the bubble of fluid that surrounds the baby. Sometimes the baby moves away from the needle as if it senses the intrusion. Other times the baby wiggles precariously close, and it seems as if the needle might prick the baby and deliver an early

warning about life's hardships, but I've never seen a baby injured.
A small amount of fluid is removed and sent in a sterile cup to the
genetics lab, where a highly trained technician cultures the cells
and then waits patiently until the cells divide.

The dividing cells, a random tangle of shapes, are captured,
fixed, stained, and studied under a microscope. Nuclei from these
cells are photographed; then individual chromosomes are cut from
the photograph and lined up in pairs, counted, and analyzed. Each
chromosome has its own unique pattern of light and dark bands,
striped like woolly-bear caterpillars. There are twenty-two pairs of
chromosomes, each packed with genes that will determine some
aspect of the baby's future, and there's one pair of sex chromosomes: XX if the child is female, XY if the baby is male. The X chromosome is the only sex chromosome women can donate. It's the
baby's father who carries both X and Y chromosomes, and therefore it is he who determines the baby's sex. If he supplies an X, the
baby will be female. If he contributes a Y, he will have a son.

A few weeks after the amniocentesis is done, the clinic receives
a glossy print of the lined-up chromosomes, looking like pairs of
bent macaroni wiggling across the page. There should be forty-six
of these squiggles, paired off, all of them whole. If a pair is dam-
aged, the twin noodles broken, or if part of a chromosome is
snapped off and attached somewhere else, something is wrong. Up
to 85 percent of early miscarriages are due to genetic abnormalities, we tell our patients. One out of 170 live newborns might have
defects, too, but often the abnormality is insignificant. Other times
the findings are classic: the extra chromosome on pair 21 that indicates Down syndrome or the extra X of Klinfelter syndrome, a
sex-chromosome deviation that occurs in about 1 out of 1,000 male
infants and results in testicular atrophy, obesity, and sometimes
mild mental deficiency. If an abnormality does occur, we draw
blood from the baby's parents, too, and a technician studies their
chromosomes as well, piecing together a tiny puzzle that will reveal the genetic history. Then the parents must decide what they
will do.

Some decide to terminate a hopeless pregnancy. Others opt to
continue the pregnancy no matter what. One couple, knowing that

their unborn girl had a deformity incompatible with life, decided to carry the pregnancy to term. If the baby were born alive, they said, they wanted no heroics, but they did want her to be fed and warmed. If by some miracle she survived, they would take her home and care for her there until she died. Laura was born two weeks before her due date, lived for three hours, and then died in her father's arms. Everyone held her, kissed her, and rubbed her, including the grandparents and three of the nurses. They wrapped her in a blanket, the pink wool tucked up high under her chin, and took her picture. People do whatever they must do.

I open the door to the ultrasound room, and Lila follows. She throws her backpack onto a chair and turns to face the ultrasound machine. We have the finest model. It sits in the corner like a fat pasha with glittering eyes, fancy buttons, and a face like a big-screen TV.

"Wow," she says. "That's it?"

"Yup. Dr. Wallace will use this transducer," I point out the broad hand piece, "to see your baby."

Ultrasounds, our patients say, are fun. They love the warm goop the doctor squishes over their bellies, they love the gentle but firm pressure of the transducer sliding over their skin, the slight heat, the small vibration. Of course, we do ultrasounds because we're interested in the basics of fetal development: Is the baby whole? Are there a functioning heart, a normal liver, a complete spinal cord? How about the mouth? Is it perfect all around, or is there a cleft, an opening that runs from lip to nostril? But our patients simply want to see their babies whole and healthy, tumbling obliviously under the pulsing probe, their images swimming close to the monitor as if they might peer out at us.

The ultrasound also gives us an opportunity to date the pregnancy and calculate when the baby is due. We compare the ultrasound measurements with the baby's age based on the mother's last normal menstrual cycle. Sometimes those two markers are right on the money and the baby is exactly as far along as the menstrual dating would suggest. Or it's way off, the baby either much bigger or much smaller. Some women don't remember the date of their last period. They don't keep track of recent or skipped cycles,

and when they discover they're pregnant, they can't answer our
question, "What was the first day of your last period?" Like Lila,
maybe, they don't keep track because they think pregnancy is
something that happens to other people.

Lila squares off in front of the ultrasound, arms akimbo, head
cocked, as if she were about to challenge a girl from a rival gang.

"So," she says, flipping one hand in the machine's direction.
"Can this doctor see if it's a boy or a girl?"

"It's probably too early, but if he does, he'll let you know."

I hand her a sheet. If her child is a boy, the external organs may
be recognized, but female genitalia lag a bit behind, both exter-
nally and internally. And sometimes, early on, a female's vulva can
be mistaken, on the ultrasound, for testicles. I don't tell her that
this doctor's so good he can trace the tiniest vessels through a
baby's heart and count the pearly bones in a baby's fingers. If any
doctor can discover the baby's sex, it's he.

Unlike Lila, our pregnant teenagers most often want boys. Few
of them know that it's the man who determines the unborn child's
sex. Sometimes, when a woman's partner learns that the baby is a
girl, he glares at her. That's when I love to explain how the system
works: how it was *his* sperm that determined the sex; how, if he's
unhappy, he has only himself to blame.

"Well, if he can't see today, he'll have to do another one later."
Lila huffs and her keys rattle. "Charles wants a girl, you know."

"Yeah, so you told me a few weeks ago. For starters, let's hope
for a healthy baby." I hesitate at the door. "Slip off your jeans, and
we'll be right back."

Lila shrugs and tosses her head. As I close the door, I hear her
start to hum. She's still humming, a thin wire of sound, when I
come back with the doctor.

"Lila, this is Dr. Wallace." Lila barely nods. She's undressed
with the sheet opened over her, already a pro at being examined.
She looks at me, so I move closer to her side.

"OK, Lila, let's go." Dr. Wallace extends the bottom of the table,
and Lila slides back. I tuck Lila's sheet down until her pubic hair is
just visible, then flick off the lights. The room settles peacefully
around us, and the monitor screen glows, reminding me of those

long-ago summer nights when I was a kid and my parents allowed me to stay outside until the first hundred stars blinked into view.

Dr. Wallace pushes a few buttons, and a band of static rolls down the screen over and over. He squirts a mound of warm lubricant over Lila's belly, plows the flat transducer head through the goop, and begins rotating his wrist to guide the probe. The static spreads out to become dense areas of gray and lighter gray, like the pattern on a TV before a video begins.

Dr. Wallace is intent, his hand maneuvering forward and back over Lila's belly as if he were casting a spell. When he leans close to the monitor, a silvery crescent appears around his gray hair and his features transform into shadow. A turn of his wrist, and a bright area appears on screen. Inside it, a small fetus squirms around like a salamander. In the center of this salamander there's a pinpoint flicker—the fetal heart that's beating 150 times a minute, about 80 times a minute more than it will beat when this baby is an adult.

We're all quiet. Lila watches the screen. Some mothers cry or laugh or say "Ahhhhhh" when they first see their babies, the fuzzy shape of the fetus, the big head and the stubby limbs. But Lila studies the monitor without expression.

"Lila, look," I say. "That's your baby." Dr. Wallace nods, taps his finger against the glass.

"Here's the heart," he says. He reaches up and presses a button, and there's a pause, then a whir, then a glossy picture emerges.

"Can I have a picture?" Lila asks.

"Sure," he says, and pushes the button a second time.

He taps the screen again. "The spine," he says. The baby's curved spine shows up like a necklace of small white interlocking beads. It is intact, the skin sealed shut around it, no sign of the spinal cord protruding through in a fleshy mass. "No evidence of spina bifida," Dr. Wallace says.

He pushes some more buttons. The screen freezes and a dotted line appears. He moves one end to the fetus's head, the other to the rump. Another button, and a list of measurements materializes alongside. Dr. Wallace hits the button again, and the fetus resumes its dance in real time.

"Thirteen weeks on the nose," he announces. "EDC December twenty-second."

Lila looks at me, and her voice comes from far away. In the dark room, I can barely make out her face.

"What'd he say?" she whispers.

"He says your baby is due on December twenty-second and that today you're exactly thirteen weeks pregnant. Just what we thought."

"Is it a girl?" She whispers again, as if afraid to disturb the doctor, whose attention is still fixed on the screen. Now he's turned on the Doppler, and blue-and-red images of the fetal blood flow appear on the screen as a fast, low *shoosh* comes from the speakers.

"I can't tell at this point, Lila. But everything looks fine." He straightens and says, "All set." I turn on the overheads, and the doctor busies himself with wiping the transducer and entering numbers on the ultrasound's keypad. I wipe the goop from Lila's belly and help her sit up. On the monitor, the last image of the baby floats in stop action, its head slightly turned so that we can see the bud of a nose and the outline of a fist as the tiny, not-quite-yet-human-looking baby sucks its thumb.

Under the fluorescent light, the three of us become strangers again. Dr. Wallace looks at Lila, and just for a second I'm embarrassed for her, and somehow for me, as if she were my child and I had neglected to tend her. A part of me, the part that even now feels inadequate before the complex knowledge of a physician, wonders if Dr. Wallace will judge my ability to care for patients based on Lila's appearance. Her hair sticks out here and there, and the almost-gone purple-green smudge under her eye—the souvenir left by Charles's fist—makes her skin look sallow. Today she's wearing six multicolored jeweled studs lined up along the curve of one ear, and the other lobe sports a single, dangling silver earring that looks, I think, like a fishing lure.

When she sits up, the key around her neck points to her belly. She looks as if she wants to say something.

The doctor hovers over Lila.

"I want you to have another ultrasound at about thirty-two weeks to see how the baby's growing. You don't smoke, do you?"

Lila's chart is open on the counter before him. He looks down at it, then up at her again as if to say "Well?"

She stares straight ahead. One shoulder lifts, a halfhearted admission. Lila reaches over to scoop up her backpack, hugs it to her.

"Can I have my picture?" she says.

Dr. Wallace hands me the picture, and I give it to Lila. She turns to smile at me and, in the glaring, impersonal clinic light, holds the grainy picture close to her eyes and studies her hazy thirteen-week-old fetus.

When the doctor leaves, I ask Lila if there's anything she wants to talk about or any questions she'd like to ask. But already whatever it was I detected on Lila's face is gone, and she's withdrawn into a country occupied only by one thirteen-week-old fetus and its mother.

"Just one more thing, Lila," I say. "Did you get a chance to show the paternity booklet to Charles?" This information explains both the rights and obligations of fatherhood in clear terms, and it includes a form for him to sign verifying his intent to support the child.

Lila fusses with her keys. She looks at me and says, "He won't sign. He ripped it up."

I look at Lila. "He ripped it up?" I count to ten. *Bastard. Bully.* "You don't have to put his name on the birth certificate if you don't want to. You also have the option of taking legal action, either to force him to support the baby or to keep him away from you." I think my voice hides my anger, but Lila studies my face so intently that I begin to wonder if I have ants crawling up my cheek or toast crumbs on my lip. I can't begin to read her look. Interest? Distrust?

"I dunno yet," she says and hoists her backpack over one shoulder. "I'll let you know."

Without another word, Lila walks out the door and down the hall. Lost in her own thoughts, she carries the small photo of her baby carefully, in both hands, as if it were made of glass.

Chapter 13

"We got one of your patients over here," the emergency room doc says when he calls. "Twenty-six-week pregnant addict with ruptured membranes. Renée Jones. You know her? I'm sending her to L and D on a stretcher."

Nina, who's the OB chief this month, asks if I want to go upstairs with her. I hurry to change into a pair of baggy blue scrubs, and the two of us fly up the metal back stairs to Labor and Delivery, my footsteps clanging, Nina's patent leather clogs making dull thuds. She's two steps ahead of me, her shiny hair jouncing up and down.

Twenty-six weeks: eleven weeks before the baby's heart, lungs, and kidneys will be developed enough to withstand delivery successfully, fourteen weeks before Renée's official due date, the last day of a forty-week pregnancy. But a baby born at twenty-six weeks might live. Maybe. If it is uncommonly strong, and if it receives the best of care. Renée's lucky; our hospital is prepared. We get preemies from all the surrounding towns, tiny almost-formed bodies with old-looking faces.

Once again, I can't help but feel that Renée has betrayed me. Right after the pepper spray incident, I'd urged her to make an appointment to begin prenatal care. I'd thought maybe *this* time she'd get it together and clean up for the sake of her baby. But she had never called, and when I tried to call her all I got was a "This phone has been disconnected" message.

"What did you expect?" Nina says to me as we emerge from the dingy stairwell into Labor and Delivery, where yellow reflections from the overhead lights dance on the hardwood floor, making my eyes burn. Huge color pictures of babies and smiling parents hang along the entranceway. Nurses sit at their station behind bowls of flowers. From up and down the hallway come the moans of women deep in labor. This is a different world from the clinic. What begins in the clinic behind closed doors, what is most hidden there—a woman's body, her sexuality, the seed that becomes a baby floating within her—is brought to fruition here, exposed for all to see. Nina pauses a moment, too, adjusting.

"Come on," she says. "You'll learn something."

Renée's stretcher, propelled through the door by two nervous-looking transporters, arrives five seconds after we do. The nurses stand up and hurry over, and we all whisk Renée into a delivery room and onto the bed, pulling off the sheets as we hoist her. She's high, sweaty and wired tight, every muscle in her body trembling. When she sees me, she closes her milky brown eyes and turns her head away. We open her legs, and there's the baby's head, just visible between Renée's thighs, pushing out along with squirts of cloudy amniotic fluid. Nina grabs a pair of gloves just in time. Skinny and limp, the baby boy slides out into her hands. Barely twenty-six weeks.

How much fight does a baby have when he's born too soon, when his lungs and heart and kidneys are barely more than a collection of cells, an imperfectly functioning set of tiny organs not yet ready to work independently? The nurses buzz around the room in their candy-colored smocks and tennis shoes. They make phone calls and page the neonatal nurse practitioners.

Nina holds the baby's glistening body in the crook of her arm. Like all preemies, his skin is thin and red, as if he'd just been dipped in scalding water. His eyelids are edematous and seamed shut. "This baby's too small," Nina says and hands the kid off to one of the two neonatal nurse practitioners who run in, out of breath. She takes the baby from Nina in one quick motion. With no time to put on a gown, she lets the sticky amniotic fluid and blood veil her arms.

The practitioner slips a thin transparent tube into the baby's throat, attaches an Ambu bag, and begins pumping air into the baby's lungs. The baby boy lies flaccid on the open warmer while the other practitioner listens to his chest with a stethoscope and then rubs him roughly with a towel, trying to stimulate even the smallest response.

Nina turns her attention to Renée. I watch everything that's going on around me, and Renée watches too. First she looks at Nina, then at me, then at the nurses.

"Whoa, hey," she says. "Boy."

"Once a druggie, always a druggie," Nina once said. Her words echo in my mind, but Nina now ministers to Renée without any hint of malice, and the neonatal practitioners are working as hard as I've ever seen them to rescue this baby boy. Renée, who has been through the system before, knows that Family Services won't allow a drug addict to take her baby home. Now she doesn't even know if her baby will live.

Nina murmurs to Renée, reassuring her that her uterus is contracting as it should, that the bleeding will stop. Renée falls silent, watching them work on her son.

The neonatal nurse practitioners talk under their breath to each other.

"This smells bad," one of them says. "His Apgar at one minute is four."

In another few minutes they will score the baby again, assessing his heart rate, breathing, color, tone, and reflexes: two points each if the heartbeat is strong, if the baby cries, if his skin pinks up, if he flexes his legs, if he coughs or sneezes. Even full-term babies rarely score a perfect Apgar of ten, but this baby is barely alive. Two points for a heart rate over 100. One point for his feeble attempts to breathe. One point for the spastic quivering of his arms.

The practitioners work their hands so fast, they blur like running water. I have seen them before, saving babies. They pump, tap, jostle, and rub, trying to convince premature infants to live.

The two women flip the baby boy around as if he were a rag doll with a painted-on face, their every move precise.

One of them leans over Renée.

"Your son is very premature," she says, "and it looks as if he probably has an infection. We're concerned that his lungs aren't mature yet. He's not breathing well on his own. We're taking him to the Neonatal Intensive Care Unit. The NICU."

She says NICU as if it were one word, *nickyou,* and then pauses, waiting for some response from this woman who stares vacantly in the direction of the warmer. Renée doesn't move, doesn't blink.

They turn, and the two of them whisk the baby away, one pumping the Ambu bag, the other guiding the warmer.

The NICU is a small, busy suite of rooms near Labor and Delivery. When a sick baby is born, he or she can be wheeled right into the NICU through an unmarked door that visitors and patients can't see. Walking into the NICU is like arriving in New York City from some isolated country. A hundred new sights and sounds assault you. Isolettes, chest-high enclosed beds in which a baby's body functions can be monitored, are stationed here and there like random islands, and above each Isolette a large, square monitor blinks its lights. Jagged lines that trace the baby's heart rate and respiratory rate ping and leap across the screen like frightened antelope. Clear plastic bags of IV fluid hang from stainless-steel hooks. Teddy bears or dolls suspended over the Isolettes sway like benevolent nannies in a desperate effort to establish normalcy. Eerily absent are the wails of crying babies.

Some babies are in oxygen hoods. Some very critical babies are still in the open warmers. Some are jaundiced, their skin a sallow yellow due to their immature liver function. Most are wrapped in gauze and tape so completely that only their birdlike heads and their scrawny feet are visible. I follow the neonatal nurse practitioners into this luminous place, curious to see what will become of Baby Boy X, just born and way too small.

When he arrives, the nurses and doctors move smoothly to his side. They've rehearsed this a hundred times. Everyone has a role, and everyone knows exactly what to do. It looks to me like a complicated, wonderful dance.

For several moments, the crowd working on this baby hides him from view, allowing me a moment to look around this strange environment. There are three other babies here, all in Isolettes. The nurses call them "houses." "Put Freddie back in his house now," a nurse might say, or "I'm going to take Alicia out of her condo."

I see two frightened people standing near one of the little houses. I suppose they are parents staying close to their baby. They don't look up when we arrive, overwhelmed with what's going on with their own child, who is frog-legged on his stomach and naked except for the giant diaper enfolding him. Their baby's back is covered with fine black hair, lanugo, the temporary growth that helps protect an unborn baby's skin from the drying effects of an amniotic fluid environment. In full-term babies, the lanugo thins by thirty-two weeks and disappears before birth. I can't read all the writing on the baby's admission card from where I stand, but the initial birth weight of 1,000 grams stands out. A dollop more than two pounds.

"And that one was a heavyweight." One of the NICU nurses, Loretta, comes over to talk to me. She and I go back a long way. I first met Loretta about twenty-five years ago, when we were new graduates lusting after the sickest patients, the most complicated cases. Loretta is still every parent's favorite nurse. She does private duty cases at night and on weekends, and sometimes, after babies go home, the parents beg Loretta to come, just one shift here and there, to help them. "After all," they tell her, "if it weren't for you we'd never be bringing Tommy home." Loretta knows it's true; she has a knack. She has arms as strong as a farmer's and an ample bosom just right for snuggling preemies.

"That's Ray," she continues, indicating the hairy frog. "He was born with a hole in his heart, no lung tissue, and a rotten attitude. But look at him now."

We watch Ray's quick, irregular breaths, and I can't imagine that this is an improvement.

"So how big is he?" I ask Loretta.

"Almost too big for this room. When he hits four pounds, he

goes to step-down. He'll go pretty soon." Next to the main NICU there's another room where the "grower" babies are stashed like pumpkins, putting on their last few pounds before going home.

Loretta introduces me around. Anne and Rosa are here, in addition to Ray and our new Baby X: two boys, two girls.

"No one knows why, but the girls always do better," Loretta says. "We get nervous when kids like this new one come in."

The cluster around Baby X has thinned, so Loretta and I go over. Loretta is my guide in this netherworld. Even though I worked in intensive care for years and in spite of my years in the operating room and on a cancer floor, regardless of all I've seen and done, this place makes me humble.

Baby X looks as fragile and evanescent as spun sugar. He'll stay on the warmer so the nurses can more easily observe him over the next critical hours. A gold, heart-shaped disk has been stuck to his chest to monitor his temperature, and a blue knit cap has been snugged onto his tiny head to help hold in body heat. His foot has been wrapped in white gauze, and a red glow throbs from beneath the layers as a tiny device attached to a toe monitors his oxygen level. An IV line called a UAC disappears into one of the two umbilical arteries. This catheter will be used to draw blood, to infuse fluids and medications, and to measure blood pressure. Another line, the UVC, travels through the umbilical vein to the baby's liver, another portal for fluid administration and pressure monitoring.

Baby Boy X weighs one pound, fifteen ounces. His skin is gelatinous and almost transparent. A net of tiny vessels cobwebs under his skin.

They've drawn his blood and attached the tube in his tiny throat to a respirator. They've already carefully poured four doses of Survanta into the breathing tube in the hope that this milkshake-thick liquid substitute for surfactant—the slippery, fatty substance that coats the airways to keep them open between breaths—will help mature his lungs. Within forty-eight hours, he'll receive his first blood transfusion, four cubic centimeters of someone else's blood. Whatever they take out in the many blood tests over the days to come, they have to put back. And Baby X, in addition to being too small, infected, and plagued by whatever else they might find, has been born addicted to heroin.

How much he will suffer depends on how much heroin Renée used and for how long. Within forty-eight hours, Baby X might develop fever, diarrhea, convulsions. The doctors and nurses will soothe his tremors and try to protect him from withdrawal by treating him with paregoric, the camphorated tincture of opium, and then they will try to wean him from that medication as well. Even so, there could be long-term effects from his exposure to heroin. As a four-year-old, Baby Boy X might be shorter than average, skinny, and unable to concentrate.

"Drugs," Loretta says. "If you want to screw up a kid, you can't beat drugs."

His limbs jerk and twitch, his blue-veined eyelids flutter. Once in a while he looks as if he wants to cry, but the tube in his throat blocks any sound. Watching his small spasms, like the involuntary leg movements made by a sleeping dog, I wonder if Baby X is dreaming.

Chapter 14

"You could be miscarrying," Yanna, one of the junior residents, says. "This early in pregnancy there isn't anything we can do to stop this process once it begins." She tells the patient to call back if things get worse, and then she hangs up.

Yanna's not my favorite resident. A California transplant with streaky hair and lots of attitude, she tells a great joke, has test scores in the top 10 percent, and is more than a little bit lazy. While the other residents pore over medical articles, Yanna thumbs through *Cosmopolitan* and plans vacations to Los Angeles. She's cursed with a photographic memory and the lack of diligence that often comes with it. She's also the only doctor I know who tries to talk patients *out* of coming in. It isn't nine o'clock yet, but already I wish a different resident were on with me today.

"Was she ever examined?" I ask, trying to piece the facts together from Yanna's side of the conversation.

Yanna licks her finger and turns a page of her magazine. "She said she'd already been seen here for her first OB visit. She started bleeding last night and went to the ER, but she didn't feel like waiting around, so she left. She couldn't have been that worried."

"Who is it?" I ask. "Anybody I know?"

Yanna looks up. "You know some kid named Lila?"

"Lila?"

"Yeah, she sounded like a teenybopper."

I pull Lila's chart and flip through to the registration sheet, but there's no phone number. My guess is that her phone's unlisted anyway, if there is one. I take out my wheel and calculate where Lila is today in her pregnancy. Fifteen weeks and six days.

Did she do too much coke? Did Charles beat her up?

Patient after patient comes in, but not Lila. The phone rings a hundred times, but it's never Lila. Yanna says, "Chill, OK? If there's a big problem, she'll land in the ER again." All I can think of is Renée and her lousy life and her born-too-soon baby. All I can picture is Lila, a baby herself, at the mercy of Charles.

About eleven-thirty, I'm in the back room ready to call the visiting nurse and ask if she'll check Main Street and the women's shelters—the only thing I can think of to do—when the phone rings. I snatch it off the hook, and this time it's Lila.

"I'm bleeding," she says. "It hurts like hell."

"Tell me what's going on."

"It's crampy all over, low down. I don't know. Sort of on the left. I can't hardly walk."

"Did anything happen?"

"Waddaya mean?"

"Were you hurt? Did anyone hit you?"

I hear Lila's little disgusted *tsk.* "No," she says.

There's a long pause.

"Did you do any drugs?"

Lila doesn't say anything. But her continued silence gives me the answer.

On the street it's common knowledge that cocaine can send you into labor, so every once in a while we get a woman who wants her pregnancy to be over, *now.* She'll smoke some coke or snort a line, then come into the hospital, suddenly in trouble. Cocaine can make the uterus go into hard, unrelenting contractions. If these contractions tear the placenta away from its uterine moorings, the engorged spiral arteries, coiled vessels nestled in the placenta, just empty and the woman hemorrhages. My guess is that Lila didn't want to end her pregnancy. She just wanted to have some fun.

Then Lila's voice again. Earnest, a little tearful.

"You know, me and Charles was celebrating the Fourth of July. I didn't do anything bad. Will my baby be OK?"

Skimming last night's ER sheet, I see that the emergency room nurse had smelled alcohol on Lila's breath when she'd come up to the desk to sign in. Her behavior in the waiting room had seemed disruptive.

I tell Lila to come to the clinic *now.* She says the bus stop is too far, she has to take a taxi but she has no money. I ask, why can't Charles drive you? She says Charles is mad at her and won't. Take a taxi, I say, we'll ask the social worker for a voucher.

By the time Lila appears, I'm tempted to let Yanna deal with her. Lila, I figure, is Yanna without the advanced education. But when Lila catches sight of me emerging from the back room, she points and calls down the hall, "I want *you* to see me."

I walk into the exam room and find her hunched over at the end of the table, her hair ratty and uncombed.

"I think maybe I'm just getting my period," Lila says by way of introduction. "Can't you get it when you're pregnant?"

"Not usually," I say.

I'm not surprised by anything a woman asks. I used to think only teenagers or undereducated women were ignorant about how their bodies worked. Now I know that most women, even highly intelligent ones, are often unable to make sense of their own physiology. Once girls were educated by a community of women, mothers and grandmothers and midwives who gathered around and celebrated the milestones of a woman's life: puberty, first menstruation, childbirth, menopause. The majority of my patients learn not from other trusted women but from harried teachers in too-full classrooms, from first boyfriends or from girlfriends who claim more experience, from magazines or cultures that convince them the ideal woman is childlike, luscious, agreeable. Some of my more progressive patients, hungry to learn about themselves, turn to the most impersonal community of all, the Internet. Imagine a woman sitting alone in front of her computer, scrolling down page after page, reading what other women have done to investigate or cure their breast cancers, their ovarian cysts, their premenstrual symptoms. The light from the screen flickers. The woman tries to link hands with an unseen female family, wanting nothing more than to talk and to listen, and by this to learn more about herself. Perhaps she does manage to gather a circle around her, but I see no true mentors for her there. Wouldn't it be better if we could once again be present for one another in the old way, face-to-face?

Lila's eyes fill with tears, and she wipes her nose with the side of her hand. "Am I gonna lose my baby?"

"I'll examine you to get a better idea of what's happening. Let's talk first. What were you doing when the bleeding started?"

"Last night me and Charles and his friends went to the fireworks. Then we went to this party. That's all." She takes her other hand and with two fingers carefully moves a stray hair away from her face. "I started bleeding when we got home."

"When did you start cramping?"

"This morning."

"How much are you bleeding?"

"Is this going to hurt the baby?" She looks like a kid afraid to tell the truth. Afraid she'll get walloped.

"Are you bleeding like a period?"

She pouts her mouth down in an I-don't-know expression.

"Did you pass anything that looked like tissue?"

"I had this clot thing." She holds up her fingers in a quarter-sized circle.

"How many pads have you used?"

"No, not like that. Like, I only saw blood when I wiped."

"How about now?"

"A little. Once this morning."

OK, so she's not exactly hemorrhaging. I begin to feel a bit more charitable. I try to remember to be kind.

"Lila, there are several things that can cause bleeding in early pregnancy. You can spot after you have sex or after a vaginal exam. Did you have intercourse last night?"

"Huh?"

"Did you have sex with anyone last night or the night before?"

Lila looks personally offended. "Who wants to do it when they're pregnant?"

"Coke can cause bleeding, too. In fact, it can cause miscarriage. How much did you use?"

"Who said I used?"

Lila's eyes overflow silently, like blue china cups.

"Why don't I examine you to see how much you're bleeding and to check if your cervix is closed."

I palpate Lila's abdomen as she lies flat on the exam table. She's not tender anywhere, just ticklish. I take a fetone and listen for the sound of Lila's baby, holding my breath until I hear it, a quick staccato gallop like the hoofbeats of a tiny horse or the rhythmic swoosh of an old wringer washing machine.

I smile and glance up at Lila, who's biting her nails. "Here's the baby's heart," I tell her.

"I knew I didn't lose the baby," she says. "So you don't have to examine me." Lila's tears have dried and disappeared without a trace, like a splash of water on a hot July day.

I have to do an exam anyway, I tell her, and when I do, I see a trace of old blood, rusty brown. Left over from last night, perhaps, or maybe not related to last night at all.

There's no new blood in her vagina. I examine her cervix, and it's closed tight.

Inside me, I feel a wave of relief. I was afraid Lila was having a spontaneous abortion, a fairly common occurrence, something that many women, myself included, have experienced. Sometimes, miscarriage is a tragedy. Other times, it seems Nature knows what she's doing.

A few years ago, I watched a miscarriage take place. The patient had come in nine weeks pregnant, cramping and bleeding, and I used cotton swab after cotton swab to clear the patient's vagina. Each time the swab emerged like a peony, the round head crimson and saturated with blood. Finally, I could see that the cervical os was open, and there, glistening in the small beam from the exam table light, was a gray mass surrounded by a crystalline, clear membrane.

My heart did a little flop. *Products of conception.* The muscular uterus had expelled the fetus, still in its jelly sack, like a cat's-eye marble. Now it had come to the end of its journey.

"I'm sorry," I said to the patient. "It looks as if you're having a miscarriage." I placed one gloved hand on the sheet wrapped around her leg for a few seconds of human contact.

Using ring forceps, I picked up a gauze and blotted more blood from her vagina. I closed the loops gently around the blob of tissue. The silver dollar–sized mass was slippery, and once, twice, it slid away. On the third try the membranous sack ruptured, and clear fluid spurted out. My heart gave another flop.

I angled the forceps in again, closed the loops around the mass, and at last lifted it gently out of the vagina. It was velvety red, part of it flat and platelike where the placental attachment had been. Without the amniotic fluid, the membrane deflated into a thin flap I could pick up and open. Somewhere inside was the minute, indistinguishable fetus, at that point looking not so much like a tadpole as a tangle of thread. Before she could see, I placed these products of conception in a plastic container and tightened the lid.

Later, the transporter came and collected our specimens, tubes and cultures that he placed into a metal rack and carried off to the lab. The little red blob in its sterile cup rode up with everything else. The pathologist scooped it out, examined the membrane, the placenta, the tiny fetus. Two weeks later his report came back and was filed in the patient's chart. That was it. No one knew why the miscarriage had occurred. The woman went home with nothing but her sorrow.

I help Lila sit up, and she scoots off the table like a woman with no time to waste.

"Take it easy for a few days, and call us right away if you begin bleeding heavily or cramping," I say. "I'm also going to talk to the ladies from outpatient Detox to set you up with an interview. The next time you come for a visit, I'd like you to give us a urine sample to check for drugs."

Lila looks at me, her face changing until it settles into a wary, impenetrable mask. "I thought you were my friend."

"I am. If you continue to use drugs, your baby could be affected. The baby could be put into foster care. It's to your advantage to prove you're clean."

"I told you I only did a little." Lila spits out the words. She forgets that she didn't tell me anything at all. "I'm no druggie."

I don't agree or disagree.

"Do you have a regular appointment scheduled?" I ask.

Lila leans against the table, tries to pull a strand of hair into her mouth. "Yeah. Next week."

"Do you have any questions for me?"

"No."

"OK. See you then. Take care of yourself."

I turn and walk out the door, and as I go I hear Lila exhale a burst of air wrapped around a single word. "Bitch."

Chapter 15

Eleanor tells me that the worst part of having abnormal Pap tests is the feeling of helplessness, as if her body were harboring hostile cells, busy at work, and there was nothing she could do to stop them. And then there are the additional tests and the endless waiting for results.

"Did I do something to cause this?" some women ask me, but I have no answers. I could say that women who don't have sex don't get abnormal Paps, but if I say that, do I blame a woman for her passion or judge her if she's had several sexual partners? Often I say that smoking is implicated in cervical cancer, as it is in so many illnesses, and if a woman smokes, I plead with her to stop. I might mention that the younger a woman is when she begins having sex and the more partners she has, the more likely she is to develop abnormal Paps. For many of our patients, that warning comes too late. Most often I discuss this with young girls during their first exam, a good time to talk about sex and disease, about pride and knowing your own mind. I tell every woman that cervical cancer, if discovered in time, can be cured.

In our clinic, cervical cancer is rare, but abnormal Paps are common. Usually the changes are transient, low-grade, and curable. Nevertheless, the visits and procedures necessary to evaluate and treat even a minor problem are exhausting, both for our patients and for us. It's difficult for a woman to understand this slow, wearing process, and it's hard for us to explain why all these tests are necessary. Time after time, a patient must come to the clinic, undress, and will herself to endure the small discomforts of the exams and the biopsies, discomforts that, when repeated so often, become almost as intolerable and defeating as chronic pain.

Eleanor's in the clinic this morning to have her colposcopy and endometrial biopsy. As I expected, she seems brave, although I know the effort this must take. She remains silent while Emily, our other chief resident, samples the lining of Eleanor's uterus with a long thin pipette. Then she swabs Eleanor's cervix with vinegar, an acidic solution that turns the abnormal cervical tissue a chalky white and fills the room with a scent reminiscent of hard-boiled eggs and paper cups of blue and lavender Easter-egg dye. Looking through the long-necked microscope, Emily takes biopsies of three suspicious-looking areas on Eleanor's cervix, three bites of tissue she deposits in a plastic vial of preservative, where they bob and float, turning the clear solution a filmy pink. Three tiny bites that, under the pathologist's expert scrutiny, might reveal cancerous cells.

I try to distract Eleanor. "How's your hubby?" I ask just as Emily snips her first biopsy. "I love your necklace," I say as Emily closes the biopsy punch a second and third time. It's one of many transgressions I can get away with as a nurse and as a woman. Would a man ever ask how a patient's "hubby" was or say "I love your necklace"?

When the procedure is over, Eleanor dresses. As she finishes arranging her shirt and shrugging on her jacket, she says to no one in particular, "Do you think everything will be OK?"

Emily says nothing, busies herself with the specimens. Her silence confirms what I suspect—that she thinks the biopsies will return with a diagnosis of cervical cancer. Then it will simply be a question of what treatment Eleanor needs and how extensive that treatment must be. She might require a loop electrosurgical excision procedure, or LEEP, a rather simple and quick maneuver we do in the clinic in which a thin wire is passed over the cervix to slice away the errant tissue and eliminate the cancer. Or she might require something more complicated, such as a cone biopsy. This surgery must be done in the OR, the patient asleep while the doctors core a larger, pyramid-shaped specimen from the cervix to remove all the abnormal tissue. Or will she require more aggressive treatment—a hysterectomy, cancer staging, chemotherapy?

Although I try to arrange my features in a pose of optimism, I have a bad feeling about Eleanor's situation. Eric, our male resident, scoffs, but the rest of us in the clinic believe in women's intuition. We get an odd premonition. Then we find the unpaid bill or we get sick or the baby falls off the bed or someone keeps calling and hanging up when we're alone.

There's another kind of intuition, too, one that most good doctors and nurses develop after many years in practice. It's as if we can smell trouble as soon as we walk into a patient's room. Sometimes, before managed care, we ordered tests based more on this special instinct than on hard medical evidence. We suspected, and sometimes discovered, certain pathologies before a patient even recognized the symptoms. "I knew it," I've heard caregivers say. "I just felt it in my bones."

Sometimes I wonder if the body of information we've come to call "women's health" is more subjective than objective. Is there a reliable group of facts and figures that are applicable to all women and therefore true for each of us? Or does every woman's individual experience in the exam room vary, thereby changing the facts? Unlike disciplines such as cardiology or pulmonology or neurology, women's health seems to me to be more fluid, ebbing and flowing differently around the ankles of each woman, the pattern of the tide forever altered by her particular presence. I like the fact that women's health seems to be a world of intuition as well as statistics—even if statistics aren't always the exact or reliable standards we'd like them to be, even if intuition, by its ephemeral nature, opens the door to anxiety.

As Eleanor leaves the clinic, she turns to stare at Emily. "So," Eleanor says. "You didn't answer me. Does it look bad?"

The suggestion of fear, thin as a gold coin, rolls in under the door.

"It's difficult to say at this point," Emily replies without look-

ing away. "Only the biopsies can tell us for sure." She squeezes
Eleanor's arm. "We'll have the results in about seven days."

The clock on the clinic wall hums. There's a persistent, dull
plong as water drips into the stainless-steel sink and bounces off
the instruments Emily has left there to soak. Rivulets of pale, rosy
blood from the tenaculums and biopsy punches trickle their way
down the drain. Claire, the nurse who assisted Emily, looks at me.

This eye language is something we nurses share with each other
and no one else, not patients or doctors or even our families—a
wordless communication that surely developed from our long history of *standing by.* Not passively waiting, but actively doing what
nurses do best: touching, listening, observing, interpreting, teaching, guiding, comforting, waiting, remembering. We stand by one
another, too.

Even though I'm a nurse practitioner and, in the hierarchy of
medicine, one step beyond a registered nurse in training and responsibility, I'm still closer to *nurse* than to *physician.* I haven't
lost that primal connection. Claire turned to me, not Emily, when
she saw Eleanor's unwavering stare and felt the loneliness inher-
ent in her words. Claire and I both saw the small, glittery fear-coin
that rolled into the room and came to rest at Eleanor's feet.

I walk Eleanor down our hallway and through the clinic door
into the lobby.

"Well, it won't be cancer," Eleanor says. "I'm sure of it." But
the pinch at the corner of her lips betrays her, and her big, swoop-
ing hands, busy at her pocketbook, seem to need something more
to do.

It's an awkward moment. What will I say if she turns to me
and asks, "What do you think?" Sometimes when patients ask me
that, I turn the question on its head. "What are you hoping I'll
say?" I reply.

"I'd like you to tell me it's not cancer," Eleanor might answer.
Or maybe "I'd like you to guarantee me that even if I have cancer,
I will still be loved."

But she doesn't ask me anything, and we stand together in silence for a moment while the hospital traffic, doctors and nurses
and men pushing patients on stretchers, swirls past. Eleanor and I

say good-bye, and I pat her arm as I turn to take off, a healthy woman striding my way through the hall to the cafeteria, my white lab coat flapping.

In one pocket, I keep the stethoscope with which I listen to patients' hearts, the wheel I use to calculate pregnancy dates, and an assortment of pens with which I write prescriptions. The other pocket holds the fat black notebook in which I've written down all the formulas, all the medication doses, all the essential phone numbers. This equipment makes me look well prepared, and sometimes I believe I am. Other days, I feel like an imposter. In spite of my collection of facts, I can't be certain of anything. No matter how strong my desire to heal, I've learned that cure is sometimes impossible.

I wait in the lunch line holding my tray, surrounded by men and women who look at home in their white coats and green scrubs. I pretend that I'm one of them.

Chapter 16

On the ultrasound, Joanna's uterus was a perfect oval. Running through the center of the oval was the thin endometrial stripe, the shadow of the uterine cavity. This lining measured at the top limit of normal, indicating that Joanna was probably about to get her period. The endometrium was velvety with the blood waiting to be shed. Her ovaries were flawless, and there was no evidence of any problems within the abdomen. Her liver, kidneys, gallbladder, and pancreas were healthy. Everything was negative. I called her with these reassuring results. She countered that in spite of those findings, her symptoms were worse, much worse. I asked if she could take time from work to come in during the day instead of in my evening clinic, just in case I wanted to pull in a senior resident. We agreed on today, and now she's here.

As soon as I enter the room, the air feels electric, as it does before a thunderstorm when the clouds are ominous and swollen. Joanna sits at the end of the table. My impulse is to say something like "Well, I hope you'll give me a chance to say hello today." With some patients, humor lightens the tension and gives us both a respite from their concerns. I don't dare try that with Joanna. Instead, I walk over, say hello, and dare to put my hand briefly on her shoulder.

"I'm glad the ultrasound was OK," I offer, "but I'm so sorry you're still having this pain." She turns her face to me, for the slightest moment accepting my empathy as if she were terribly thirsty and I'd arrived offering water. Then her expression changes, and she tries to control whatever waits inside her, brittle as tinder.

"I don't want to have sex anymore. I just *can't*. Probably because I did something stupid. Really stupid."

I remember the first words she ever said to me: "I think I'm allergic to sex." I wait a few seconds before I reply. "What's going on?"

She sits perfectly still, facing me, yet her anxiety—or is it her fear?—is palpable.

"Do you want to talk about it?" I ask.

She laughs for the first time, a brief expulsion of air. "You could say I had a one-night stand. Oh God, this was *so* stupid."

I don't say anything. This time it's my turn to continue looking at her. No expression on my face. No judgmental frown, no self-righteous smirk. Just waiting.

"There's this other guy, someone in a company I do a lot of work for. I don't know, it seemed like it just happened."

"What happened?"

"A few weeks ago . . . I met him for dinner, and then we had sex. I don't know why—maybe I thought the pain wouldn't be there with someone else. I don't know what I thought. It just *happened*."

Some women might begin to cry, but Joanna doesn't. Her eyes don't shine, her nose doesn't redden. "The pain was the same," she says. "Even worse."

I wait for her to continue. It might be kinder for me to interrupt, dismiss this as if her behavior were reasonable—a woman trying to find out what's going on with her body or a woman abandoning herself to passion. But I know that curiosity or desire didn't have anything to do with it. I think Joanna just didn't have the emotional reserve to say no.

"Now all I can think is what if this guy has something?" she says. "I've always been careful anytime I've had a new partner. You know, do they have HIV? Do they have anything else?" She expels her breath, a deep, cleansing sigh. I take a breath too. Once I took a yoga class, and that's how the teacher began the hour, with each of us taking a deep breath to bring the world whirling around us to a stop.

"I can't believe I did this to David," she says.

She lets me rest my fingers on her arm. "It's always easy to say that looking back," I offer. "But there are reasons for what we do. We just have to figure them out."

"Can you test me again for sexually transmitted diseases?" she asks. "Can you test for all of them?"

"Of course. I can also draw some blood."

"For what?"

"For syphilis, hepatitis, and HIV."

"Is there anything else? Can you test me for herpes?"

"When I examine you, if I see a blister or a lesion that looks suspicious, I can do a special culture." I wait to see if Joanna will say anything more without my asking.

Is her affair evidence of a shift in her relationship with David? If a stable partnership suddenly doesn't meet a woman's needs, the problem might be a lack of communication. One or both of the partners might feel stressed or bored or taken for granted, or any one of the hundreds of emotions that are stirred and magnified within any partnership. If Joanna could *talk* to David about her symptoms and their implications, would he be willing to support her? Or are there deeper issues for Joanna? More and more, I'm convinced that her symptoms and her behavior are evidence of a long-term problem, one that she has, consciously or unconsciously, fought to keep at arm's length. For years, she has managed to protect herself. Now her blindfold is beginning to slip.

Unable to reveal her feelings or define the source of her symptoms, Joanna has let her actions speak for her. First she started having unbearable pain with sex, then she wandered into an encounter with a new man. What Joanna's intellect wasn't able to say, her body could: Stop! Don't touch me! Look at what's going on here! Crazy relationships, sexual difficulties, and inappropriate liaisons are not the domain solely of my poor or undereducated patients.

The last time I saw Joanna, I suggested that she and David seek

therapy, but her obvious anxiety, combined with her bland willingness to be examined and exposed, stopped me from insisting. I
was afraid she would flee and never come back, refusing any help
I might provide. But today, I vow to myself, I *will* say something.

"I didn't even make him use a condom." Joanna is shaking her
head. "I didn't even ask if he had one. How," she asks, "could I be so
dumb?"

Joanna lets me examine her. I palpate her neck to search for
any swollen lymph nodes, and I look in her throat for signs of
infection—sometimes evidence of sexually transmitted diseases
lurk there, too. Her throat is slightly red. There's a velvety patch on
the left side.

"Joanna, did you take this man's penis in your mouth?" I say
this as casually as if I'm inquiring "Does that recipe require two
cups of sugar or only one?" Sometimes I have to say things that
might shock a patient or give her pause, but I'm not asking frivo-
lously. I'm an ally, not an interrogator.

She answers, "No, I didn't."

"Have you noticed any change in your vaginal secretions?"

"I noticed some yellow discharge," she says. "That really got me
worried."

"I see," I reply. Then I give my standard talk, as if my patter
could make this encounter seem like any other. "It's normal for
women to have some vaginal discharge. Sometimes it's white and
dries yellow on your underpants. Sometimes it's clear and viscous.
It depends on where you are in your cycle."

Often women are surprised to learn that they are *supposed* to
have vaginal discharge, that its presence and character are medi-
ated by our hormonal cycles, and that some women produce more
discharge than others. That it's a concern only if the discharge
itches or burns, if it's clotted and thick as it can be with yeast, or
greenish or gray with a fishy odor, an indication of trichomoniasis
or a bacterial vaginosis. Too often, women detect normal discharge
and think they have an infection, immediately douching or treating themselves with an over-the-counter cream. Sometimes getting
rid of the discharge becomes an obsession, leading to a cycle of irritation, medications, clinic visits, and frustration.

But when a woman takes a new partner, as Joanna has, any change in discharge takes on another dimension as well. Even the cleanest man, the most pristine woman, might harbor sexually transmitted infections. I learned that when I met Carole. She was dressed in a jersey skirt and scrunched-down socks, and she came into the clinic at the end of a semester break, ready to return to college and intercollegiate hockey. She'd had two sexual partners in her eighteen years, both fraternity men. I had to tell her that her HIV screen was positive.

I say this to my patients all the time: *You can't tell if people have a sexually transmittable disease just by looking at them.* More than twelve million women a year in the United States are affected by sexually transmitted diseases. Joanna is worrying that she is one of them.

"How about if I had something like chlamydia?" she asks. "Wouldn't I know it by now?"

"You might not. Sometimes women experience increased discharge and burning, other times there isn't much in the way of symptoms."

I do the cultures, and as I do I look for any evidence of purulent cervical discharge. I see nothing out of the ordinary. I do a wet mount and find no evidence of yeast, bacteria, or trichomonads.

After she's dressed, I draw Joanna's blood. Her vein, engorged by the pressure of the tourniquet, is plump and thick. When my needle tip punctures it, a single drop of blood springs out and trembles on her skin. I draw several tubes, vials the color of amethyst, garnet, ruby: HIV, pregnancy, hepatitis screen, syphilis. The tubes clatter into the wire basket.

"Thank goodness for that great vein," I say, and she responds, her face for a moment becoming animated, as if she'd almost forgotten what was on her mind, as if she'd awakened one morning and for that instant forgotten the troubles that had kept her awake the night before. Then she remembers.

"I don't know what to do," she says.

I recognize an opportunity and take it.

"I'm concerned that your symptoms may be related to some sexuality issues. Even though you just started having pain recently, the cause of the pain may be something long-standing. I don't have an answer for you, Joanna. There might not be an easy answer. I can certainly make sure that your body is healthy and that you have no infections or physical reasons for pain, but a therapist would be better able to help you explore some other issues. To find out what else is going on."

I finish my proposal rather lamely, my voice hesitating after "going on," as if I might keep on talking and come up with what those "other issues" might be.

"I remember, too, that you said David was willing to go into counseling with you. It sounds as if he'd be very supportive."

Joanna says nothing, but shakes her head no. Her expression says, "No, not me. No, I don't want to." Her rigid shoulders say, "If I go, I might find out what I don't want to know."

"I'll call you with the GC and chlamydia results in two days," I say. "I won't have your HIV results for about a week, and I'd like to see you in person to give you those."

Even when an HIV test is negative, it's better to say that face-to-face. Better to have another chance to talk about the patient's risks and fears, real or imagined.

Joanna says, "I was hoping *you* would have some suggestions on how I could make myself, you know, be more normal again. I feel comfortable with you." She looks tired and, in spite of her sophistication, quite bewildered. Joanna is finally beginning to feel at ease with me, and here I am asking her to see someone else, to say it all again. To start at the beginning.

Like so many others, Joanna's a single women at the beginning of a new millennium. In addition to whatever her deeper issues might be, she lives in sexually turbulent times. I was a young divorced mother in the late 1960s and early 1970s, decades of change that raged all around me with free love and marijuana and *Hair* shocking everyone on Broadway and the Beatles and Janis Joplin and outdoor rock concerts. When I worked as an aide and later, when I was a student on the hospital wards, I grew accustomed to discovering interns and nurses in midembrace behind a linen closet door or in a patient's empty room. But there was a certain innocence then that I recall as well: flower power, a generous, loving undercurrent as my baby-boomer generation discovered what we thought was a way to be unlike the regimented, overly scheduled parents who'd given us bottles according to Dr. Spock's strict rules and taught us to be polite and accommodating no matter what. We'd never heard the words "HIV" or "AIDS." In the 1970s, that virus was only lurking. The worst gynecologic event we faced was unexpected pregnancy. I remember one friend, her long hair braided with beads, her smock dress expanding with her belly. No longer hustled off to give birth secretly, as a few teenage girls in my high school had been, this woman cherished her love child and enlisted whole groups of friends as surrogate aunts and uncles.

When I look at Joanna now, that time and that sensibility seem very long ago, its many imperfections—risk, violence, drug abuse, war—distorted by memory. Today, the world of dating, sex, and relationships is a more perilous place.

I give her the names and phone numbers of the hospital's mental health clinic and of two social workers who have private practices and who might consider reducing their fees. I urge her to call one of them. I'm not a therapist, but I've discovered a lot about Joanna, more than she thinks she has revealed. After her first visit, I wasn't certain what was going on with her. At her second visit, my anxiety escalated in her presence, and my intuition kicked in, suggesting a diagnosis that I still wasn't sure of. Now I am.

Joanna doesn't look at the paper I hand her but folds it into her pocket as if, out of sight, the names might disappear and their implications could be ignored. I give her an appointment card for my evening clinic, too, and on the top I write, "Just to talk."

Chapter 17

As Renée and I walk together down the hall toward the NICU, I no-
tice that our heads are about the same height, bobbing up and
down as we go, I in my flats and Renée shuffling along in those
stretchy sock slippers they give out in hospitals. It's been several
weeks since her baby was born—last week she finally named
him Marvin—and now she's allowed to visit him whenever she
wants, but only with supervision. She's still a patient on the detox
floor, and as we get off the elevator I notice that she looks a little
blurry, as if someone has rubbed out her body's sharp outline.
Methadone can do that, and she's on big doses. Marvin's detoxing,
too, a process that could take weeks. Until then, he's the hospital's
youngest addict.

We turn down the long corridor toward the NICU, past the
dusty artificial plants and the generic watercolors that decorate the
walls.

"So," Renée says.

I look in her direction.

"So you think this'll work or what?" she asks.

Renée couldn't find anyone else to supervise her visit today, so
she asked me if I'd go with her. I reluctantly agreed. Today's a special day, and, she'd pleaded, she really wanted to be here. Today

they're going to take Marvin off the respirator and see if he can breathe on his own.

"I think it will be OK, Renée," I say. "And if he doesn't do well, they can always try again in a day or so." I bring my hand up to touch her arm, not because I want to but because I think I should. Her blue-and-white-striped robe feels rough and overstarched.

We walk through the sliding doors into the NICU, and Renée pulls me right over to Marvin. One of the nurses has written "MARV" on a blue-edged card taped to the side of his plastic house. Inside, he looks like a lump of receiving blankets and plastic wiring. In his short life, he's been through a lot. A CAT scan of his brain was normal, but a cardiogram and sonogram, Loretta told me, revealed a patent ductus arteriosis. A "hole" in his heart.

Like all babies before birth, Marvin received oxygen not by breathing but from his mother's blood as it circulated through the placenta. His oxygenated blood then traveled to the right side of his heart, where it was pumped through a short tube, the ductus arteriosis, directly into his aorta, bypassing Marvin's inactive lungs and rushing to his various organs. When a baby is born and takes his first breath, this ductus arteriosis normally closes. From that moment on, blood flows from the right side of the heart to the lungs, where it picks up oxygen, then back through the left side of the heart and out the aorta, speeding its precious cargo to all the cells of the body. In preemies born before the lungs are ready to work, this automatic closure doesn't always occur, so the ductus remains open, or patent.

Marvin is receiving doses of Indocin, a medication related to ibuprofen that helps close the ductus. That's why we tell expectant mothers not to take Advil or Motrin or any other ibuprofen in the last half of their pregnancy. If they do, we worry that their unborn baby's ductus might begin to close prematurely, shunting blood to the lungs before the baby's able to breathe. "Marvin's lucky," Loretta had said to me. "We caught it in time."

Since Marvin was born, he has had his own nurse every day, a one-on-one intense relationship that lasts for the eight-hour shift. Four days a week it's Loretta. Three days a week it's someone else.

The nurses take Marvin's pulse, blood pressure, and respiratory rate every hour. They slip catheters into his breathing tube and suction out the thick, gluey secretions that keep his immature lungs "stiff." They stand and stare at him through the glass, wondering if all their work will pay off. When he gains a fraction of an ounce, they celebrate.

"I hear he's doing really well," I say to Renée.

She stands mutely waiting for the doctors and the neonatal nurse practitioner to arrive, until one of the lights over Marvin begins to flash and the warning bells ding. Then Renée looks about in desperation.

"Over here," she calls, waving her arms at the nurses. "Alarm going off!"

The nurses don't seem to hurry, yet they arrive swiftly. They put on gloves, pick Marvin up, and unwrap his gauze feet. They readjust the tiny, tiny catheters that invade his tiny, tiny veins, and the chiming stops. They smile at Renée and rub her arm in assurance. They whisper to me that if she could only wean from the methadone, she could pump her breast milk and save it for Marvin. Who knows, it might help. Behind her back, angry that all their efforts might be wasted, the nurses say, "She shouldn't be allowed to take this baby home."

After he was born, Marvin spent several days lying blindfolded under a special spotlight. Born too soon, he lacked the enzymes necessary to break down one of the chemicals released from his used red blood cells, so this indirect bilirubin built up in his skin. Marvin glowed like a buttercup. The doctors ordered phototherapy, a method discovered years ago by nurses when they noticed that premature babies placed by a sunny window did not become as jaundiced as the other babies. Now "bililights" are used to help a baby's body eliminate the stubborn indirect bilirubin. Renée thought it was all pretty funny. "Hey, my daisy boy," she laughed.

Marvin is no longer yellow. Now he's that odd, born-too-early pink and as skinny as Renée. Sometimes he opens his eyes. They're cloudy and somber, and they swim around like two sunfish in a dirty pond. He's still getting paregoric to quiet his withdrawal seizures, and he's still fed through a tube with a buttery fluid that, for a while, rivaled his skin tone. Every day, Renée has come down from the seventh floor to see him. In the beginning, the nurses were surprised that she visited so often. A few said she probably didn't care about the baby at all but only wanted to get away from the restrictions of the detox ward. Perhaps. But now, when I watch Renée as she watches Marvin, I believe that she really wants to be here. Maybe she sees that he's a fighter, as she is. Maybe she thinks she's the only one in the world who loves him. Maybe she thinks he's the only one in the world who might love her. Whatever the reason, her baby's suffering has become her own.

A neonatologist arrives with Loretta and one of the neonatal nurse practitioners. Renée and I stand aside while they crowd around Marvin's house, creating a great white wall we can't see beyond. Around us, the NICU is unusually quiet.

"Oh, hey," Renée says and crushes my hand. "What if it don't work? Will he die?"

"If he can't breathe on his own, they'll put him right back on the breathing machine. They won't let him die. They said he's really strong."

"What if it don't *ever* work?"

"It will. Loretta says he's a tough little guy."

"Jeez," Renée repeats, over and over, while the doctor adjusts some dials on the respirator, then leans over the baby with a stethoscope. Renée grips my arm with both hands so hard it feels like a combination of need and punishment. Her nails dig half-moons into my flesh, and she tightens her fists until I have to shake her away.

"Come on, Renée. Let's move to where we can see so we don't have to imagine what's going on." I drag her over until we can see the baby's blue-stockinged head behind the white backs of the medical team. Marvin's pigeon chest pants up and down. The doctor pulls the narrow breathing tube from the baby's throat, and Marvin coughs and wheezes with a small, pathetic sound.

The lights and alarms begin to chime and ding, and Loretta reaches over and snaps them off. Then she turns off the respirator. The machine sighs, a long sizzle of air, and the bellows collapse and stop. The only sound is Marvin's puny huffing. The spotlight above us beats down as if it were high noon. The lights are always on in the NICU. There's no bedtime, no time to rise and shine.

"Hey hey," Renée says. "Is he breathin'?"

"Looks like he's doing fine. They'll be keeping a close eye on him."

Part of me cheers Marvin on, my heart breaking to see this innocent human thing that struggles so bravely. Another part of me is hardened against Renée and, by association, against Marvin. I tell myself that I don't care much about either one of them. Marvin's success is, at best, tentative. If he does manage to stay off the respirator, he'll have lots of "As" and "Bs," periods of apnea when he will forget to breathe or episodes of bradycardia, times when his heart rate will drop. Most of the time, he'll remember to breathe on his own. When he doesn't, a nurse will flick his foot or rub his back, reminding him that he's alive and has work to do. Imagine how attentive that nurse must be—a hundred times more present than a drug-addicted mother.

Renée stares at Marvin, but her fingers are busy picking at her skin. Once in a while she wipes her nose or tugs at her bathrobe or looks around the room as if she sees roaches skittering across the ceiling. We wait together like this, Renée's vibrations the only disturbance around Marvin's Isolette. Eventually, the medical crowd clears and only Loretta stands guard over Marvin's shallow, flickering breaths.

"Hey, I almost forgot," Renée says to me. "Look what I brought."

She holds out a crumpled black-and-white photo. "A picture of myself. Can I give it to him?"

Loretta says, "Sure you can," and she raises the plastic crib top and motions Renée over. Renée starts to prop the photo in one corner, then changes her mind and places it carefully in front of her son's face, just in case he might open his eyes. In the photo, Renée is sitting on a man's lap and waving a cigarette overhead. The smoke from the cigarette curls around her face and billows behind her like a cape. The man's face is turned away, as if he isn't paying Renée any attention.

I wonder, when she looks at the photo now, how she interprets his half scowl, his preoccupation with something or someone just out of the frame. Why did she choose this picture anyway? Because she's smiling? Because the man in the picture might be Marvin's father? Because this is the only photograph she has of herself?

Loretta guides Renée's hand to help her stroke her son's cheek. Loretta doesn't think bad thoughts about Renée. She believes in positive energy. Anyway, she has her own past to deal with: a boy she gave up for adoption and a few run-ins with abusive boyfriends along the way. Loretta has told me how she talks to Renée about recovery, about how her life could be better in the future.

"Look at me," she says.

Loretta winks at Renée. "Come back soon and I'll teach you to kangaroo," she says.

"To *what?*"

"Kangaroo. You unwrap the baby and hold him against your bare skin. He feels your breathing and hears your heartbeat, and that helps him to regulate his own."

"Ha," Renée says. "Yeah, OK." Just the thought of having to hold Marvin with all his wires and catheters makes her shudder. I imagine Renée cradling her son's naked scrawny body against her bare chest as if he were a tiny joey secure in his mother's pouch. Maybe that simple act will be the miracle necessary to jog Renée out of her hellish existence.

She turns to look at me. "OK, OK, time to split," she says, and walks away.

I've used up more than my lunch break. Most of the residents are busy in surgery today, so when I get back to the clinic there will be a bunch of restless patients waiting, anxious to have their exams and be done with it. So why, I ask myself, am I doing this?

Like an answer, the image of Renée timidly stroking Marvin's cheek comes to my mind. Renée's almost out the double doors. I hurry after her.

Chapter 18

I flip through Lila's chart, wheel out her dates, and realize that her pregnancy is half over. I haven't seen her for a while. One week she came in while I was on vacation; the next visit Nina saw her. I still have mixed feelings about Lila's commitment to this pregnancy; nevertheless, I'm fond of her. She's half streetwise and half innocent, and her bumbling determination reminds me of the earnest, as well as the dangerous, mistakes I've made along the way. When I see Lila, her shaggy hair and her untied shoes, I think of myself, newly divorced with no money for clothes, standing in line in the consignment shop but charging a stereo on my one overburdened credit card so I could listen to the Moody Blues after work and pretend that our family was like all the others. When I see Lila, seemingly so disconnected from all that's going on about her, I remember when I was so desperate for money I pawned a necklace my mother had given me for my sixteenth birthday.

It was one perfect sapphire, my birthstone, surrounded by tiny old-fashioned diamonds and suspended on an antique gold chain. When my mother gave it to me, she talked about its history, how it had been passed on from mother to daughter for three generations, a family tradition. But now I was twenty-three, on my own, and I needed money to pay my rent more than I needed this delicate necklace. I had two young children, two jobs, and nowhere else to go. The man at the pawnshop gave me twenty-five dollars, a windfall. Months later, when I'd managed to scrape together enough money, I returned to the pawnshop to buy back my necklace. As I walked into the narrow, dusty storefront, I saw my family heirloom in a smudgy glass case. The price tag said twelve hundred dollars. When I offered my savings, the shop owner said, "You must be kidding." I reminded him that he'd paid me only twenty-five dollars for it, and anyway, I screamed at him, it's *my* necklace. He laughed and put his face right into mine. *You don't get how this works, do you?*

After I was divorced, I lived with my kids in a no-frills apartment, four small rooms stuck together like four drab blocks from my children's toy box. A friend who lived in an identical brick building across the parking lot invited me over one evening. "Come on," Beverly said. "Dave and Cathy are here. Come have some fun." I had been working and going to school full-time forever. I was tired and frustrated, despairing that I could never pull myself and my children out of poverty's steep-sided pit. All I wanted was to get away, just for a while, from such overwhelming responsibility. In the background, I could hear records blasting in Beverly's living room: Led Zeppelin. Jefferson Airplane.

My kids were asleep, motionless in their beds, their breath barely stirring the air around them. Beverly said, "Leave them there." She had a plan. When we were through talking, we didn't hang up. I put the black phone receiver in my children's doorway, stretching the cord and hooking the handset over a chair. I stood watching them for a long time. Their chests rose and fell quietly. Once in a while their eyelids fluttered and their hands quivered, as if they were looking at me and trying to wave from the blue cave of their sleep. Then I turned, locked the door, pocketed the key, and ran over to Bev's.

For two hours, I sat with her phone pressed to my ear, listening for a groan or cry that would send me sprinting the few hundred feet back to my apartment. But all I heard was silence, a profound nothingness. Separated from my children by the dull gray parking lot and the narrow cement halls, I listened to hear evidence that they even existed, any sleep sound that would reinforce the reality of their presence. I stayed, phone to one ear, Grace Slick and her band high and wailing in my other ear.

What if there had been a fire? What if someone had broken into my apartment—not an uncommon occurrence in that neighborhood—and found my son and daughter? When I look at Lila, I remember being alone and poor and at my wit's end. When I look at Lila, her swollen belly, her thin lips, her jangle of earrings and chains, I remember something a great poet once told me. "Poems that are too perfect," he said, "like lives that are too ordered, lack the human mistakes that make them real." Because I never forget the reality of what I've experienced, I can forgive many of the mistakes I see my patients make. Because I know that I am a different person now, I trust that they, too, will change; that the girl Lila is now is not the woman Lila will become.

———

Nina's note from the last visit says that Lila seemed depressed. When Nina asked her, Lila denied being suicidal. "No thoughts of killing or hurting herself," Nina wrote. "Still happy about being pregnant. Denies further drug use." She had walked Lila over to Detox, where a social worker was waiting to interview her. Then the social worker had sent her home. Home to Charles and his mother.

Apparently, Charles's first girlfriend had had a fight with his mother and moved out, taking their son, Tyler, with her. So Lila had left the apartment she shared with another teenager and moved in with Charles and his mother, taking the girlfriend's place. In addition to everything else, Lila, back in the sack with Charles, had contracted chlamydia. Nina had treated her with four big pills and given her a telephone number Charles could call for free medication.

I square my shoulders and knock on Lila's door.

"Hello, Lila," I greet her, and she turns at the sound of my voice.

Her hair is just barely red-tipped, cut very short with drab blond roots almost halfway down to the straight ends. A halfway day.

"Davis." I see she's taken to calling me by my last name. "I haven't seen you for ages. I thought you quit!"

I smile at this and stand in front of her, clasping her chart. The last time I saw her, she called me a bitch. I guess she has forgiven me.

"Lila, you're halfway through the pregnancy today. Congratulations. Four and a half months!"

Lila's face darkens. "I thought I was six months."

I show her my wheel and explain the forty weeks of pregnancy, how that's nine and a third months. How twenty weeks is halfway through a forty-week pregnancy. Lila hisses like a snake.

"God, I thought this was almost over." She looks into the space between us.

Lila has entered that long dry spell of pregnancy. The excitement of the first few weeks is over, gone with the flurry of blood tests and cultures, with the reassuring ultrasound that checked the baby's size and confirmed the due date, with the triple screen test that examined Lila's blood to see if her unborn baby was at risk for Down syndrome or spina bifida. It's eight weeks until the next blood test, fourteen weeks until the next vaginal exam. These are boring visits and boring times: weight, blood pressure, urine dip, listen for the fetal heart, measure the pregnant belly. At this point, Lila is able to feel her baby move in intermittent taps and flutters. The big kicks will come later. And although her waist has thickened, losing the gentle curve it had before, she still doesn't *look* pregnant. No one looks at her, then offers to hold the door. No elderly grandmas have asked if they can rub her belly. It's like a long stretch on the highway without trees or gas stations, without exits.

"How are you feeling?" I ask, and Lila rolls her eyes. It's plain that we have to reestablish our relationship. Oh, what a few weeks can do.

"The nurse's note says everything looks fine today," I tell Lila. "Your blood pressure's great, no bacteria or protein in your urine.

You've been gaining just the right amount of weight. And your drug screen last visit was clean. Good job!"

She rolls her eyes again, but this time she rubs her barely protruding abdomen and smiles.

"I weigh a ton," she says. "Look at the size of this kid."

I pull out the foot extension, and Lila lies back. She billows the white sheet to cover her legs and pulls down her stretchy shorts to expose her abdomen. I use the side of my hand to find the top of her uterus. First my fingers move against the pliant give of her skin, then they meet the upper edge of the fundus, a firm round resistance right at her belly button. Just where it should be.

"Perfect," I say. "See, here's the top of the uterus. All this is baby down here." I sweep my hand over the convex bowl of her abdomen. "Do you feel the baby move?"

"Hmm. I think a little. Like a tickle."

"Just wait, pretty soon you'll be feeling big kicks."

I open the lubricant and squeeze some on the fetone. As I glide the probe over her belly, we hear Lila's heart, a slow *shu shu,* and then the quick, galloping sound of the baby's heart, *du du dut, du du dut, du du dut.* Lila giggles.

"Can I have another ultrasound to see if it's a boy or a girl?" She looks at me for the first time this visit. It's a familiar request.

"We're going to do another ultrasound when you're thirty-two weeks. Then, if the baby's cooperating, we might be able to tell."

I help Lila sit up. She scrunches her nose. A few seconds of silence pass, but it seems like several minutes.

I know I could end the visit here, give Lila a two-week return appointment, tell her to call if there are any problems, and then be out the door. Part of me wants to do that. It's almost time to close the clinic, and it's so warm outside that all the patients have come in wearing shorts and sleeveless T-shirts. But if I leave now, I'll feel guilty.

"So, Lila, I hear you're living with Charles and his mom. How's that going?"

Lila's lips tighten, and she begins twirling the ends of her hair. "OK," she says.

I don't say anything, just keep looking at Lila. I tell myself I have the upper hand here. I can wait comfortably.

"OK," she says again and readjusts her sock, reties her sneaker. Her nails are bitten down to the ends of her fingers.

I shift my weight to the other foot. Maybe, I think, maybe things are really looking up.

"Except," she begins, readjusts the other sock, reties the other sneaker.

I wait. "Except?"

"Except maybe this pregnancy was a big mistake." She looks surprised at the sound of her own voice. Then she can't stop, and the words spill out around us.

"I mean, if he had this other kid already, why did he get *me* pregnant? Then he has *her* living with him while he's partying with *me*? Then she has a fight with his mother and they throw her out and he's like all broken up so he asks me *now* will I stay with him? You know? And I was happy where I was. Now my roommate already rented my half of the apartment so I can't go back and it's like all day his mother is telling me what to do and how I should name the baby and how *she* wants it to be a boy."

Lila catches her breath. All of her anger at Charles is right there festering like a boil, a pocket of infection begging to be lanced.

"And so there I am and he's like goin' out at night with his friends and he gives me that *infection,* so I have to take these huge pills that make me feel *sick,* and he took *his* time getting *his* medicine."

I sit down on the stool and roll back.

"I'm sorry. It sounds like you're miserable." I realize this is the understatement of the day. I also realize Lila has no other place to live.

"I mean, I love him and everything, and he's really *happy* about the baby, he says, but I mean, if I knew . . ." Lila shrugs. "You know."

"That must have been really hard for you, having to move in after Charles's girlfriend moved out and all."

"Yeah, she's a bitch, you know. She's calling him again, and he sneaks off and calls her. You know what he tells me? 'No, it wasn't her on the phone, it's none of your business who I talk to anyway.' I know it's her."

"I'm sorry, Lila." Pause. Wait a few beats. "What do you think you'll do?"

The question hovers between us. Doing something to change her life is a new concept for Lila. She looks at me as if I'm deaf, stupid, or impossible.

"Me and Charles are going to move out and get our own place."

I can see Lila picking out curtains and tablecloths, buying ant traps and dish detergent. Playing house.

"I see. Before the baby comes?"

"I guess. I mean, we've got to save some money, and his mother makes him pay most of his state check to her and I got to give her rent, too, so most of mine's gone. So it's hard." Lila's face lights up. "But I got a crib picked out. We think the baby should have her own room, you know? Like, if we call it a *her* maybe it'll be a her."

There's so much magical thinking in the air I can barely breathe.

"Well, I hope things work out for you, Lila. I wonder if our social worker can give you any help with finding an apartment." I hope Lila might agree to see the social worker again today. Maybe Meg can work on self-esteem and an apartment at the same time.

Lila gets that blank look. How dare I? I've just suggested that she turn fantasy into reality by taking some action, and that's enough to turn her to stone. Maybe, too, she knows that increasing her dependence on Charles could mean trouble down the road. Maybe she knows if she stops telling herself how much she loves Charles and how much he loves her, she'll really feel alone.

"I don't like her," Lila says, dismissing Meg with a gesture. "She'd just as soon lock me up and take my baby away."

"I think she wants you to have your baby and then be able to take care of it."

Lila sighs, a big, heavy sigh. "Can I go? Are we done? I got stuff to do."

Maybe I've come too close to the bone. Or maybe Lila's just bored. She looks around and gathers her backpack, her soda can, a bundle of papers from the financial counselor that she has to take to the state assistance office downtown, a plastic beeper that she hooks onto her belt, and a bunch of keys so huge I wonder if she has collected keys all her life. Maybe one of them belongs to a house where Lila used to feel safe.

"Yup, we're all finished. Let me know if you'd like to see Meg next time. We'll see you back again in two weeks."

Two weeks. To Lila, an eternity.

She's already out the door and down the hall, crowding up to Kate's desk, where she sees a friend. The two of them squeal, juggle their bundles of papers and appointment cards, touch each other's stomachs and push against each other, shoulder to shoulder, tossing their heads and laughing out loud like children set free in a playground. Then the girls turn, and I see them face on—the bloated circle of their bellies, their empty eyes.

Chapter 19

The pathology conference room is long and narrow with a pol-
ished oak table in the middle. Once a month, the attending physicians gather around the table with the two chief gynecological
residents to present cases. The rest of us—nurse practitioners, residents, and students—sit in folding chairs set up along the walls.
As we concentrate on the pull-down screen at the far end of the
room, shelves crowded with leather-bound books stand guard behind us. These volumes hold the pathology reports of all the cells
and all the organs harvested from patients during various tests and
operations since the hospital opened. What's missing from these
reports are the patients themselves: what they looked like, what
made them laugh, who desired them. Somewhere on these shelves
is the account of Eleanor's Pap tests and biopsies, illustrated by all
the colorful slides the pathologist made. But nowhere does it say
"Kind teacher" or "Woman whose hands fly up like chickadees."

The results of Eleanor's colposcopy biopsies were not good.
The pathologist detected evidence of a tiny area of cancerous
cells—carcinoma in situ—the early changes that might, untreated,
progress to invasive cervical cancer. The next logical step in the sequence is for Eleanor to have a cone biopsy, an even larger cervical
sampling done not in the clinic but with a scalpel in an operating

room. Emily told Eleanor the colposcopy results. She also said she wanted to run her case past a panel of experts. Emily said Eleanor had nodded and set her mouth in a tight, straight line.

Here in Tumor Board, I'm right in the middle of the old boys' network and light-years away from the friendly atmosphere of the clinic. This pathology conference room filled with cancer specialists seems like a military tribunal. The unspoken hierarchy of command is so ingrained and so irrefutable that it's almost comical. If a resident or student should sit by mistake in the wrong chair— especially the one at the head of the room that the chief oncologist occupies—the moderator taps the table with his glasses and clears his throat until the offender backs away. If the pathologist finishes discussing a slide and then raises his arm to signal "Lights on" but the secretary doesn't see his gesture, we all sit there in darkness, no one willing to get up and flip the switch, thereby confirming his or her inferior status.

The oncologist and the head pathologist are the generals, and the radiologist is second in command. The gynecological surgeons come next, foot soldiers who have done time in the trenches. There are always visiting dignitaries, too, this time an oncology fellow from New York, a hematologist, and the gynecologists whose patients are being discussed. The OB-GYN residents are here to learn. It's their job to present any patients diagnosed with gynecological cancers during the past few weeks and to answer the barrage of questions the experts will throw at them, testing how well the residents have done their studying. The pathologist shows slides of the patient's Pap tests or biopsies. Everyone then discusses which follow-up treatment should be done, each doctor favoring his own discipline. The oncologist votes for chemotherapy, the radiation oncologist quotes the statistics on the efficacy of whole-pelvis radiation, and the surgeons wonder if enough tissue was removed.

There are two secretaries, one who takes minutes and another who jumps up to turn the lights off when the slides are shown and on again afterward. The junior residents and various medical and nursing students sit and listen where I do, on the periphery. In order to see the slides, we move forward and backward in our folding chairs, trying to peer over the generals' heads.

Today, Nina will present the first case, and Emily will go next and talk about Eleanor. Nina's dressed in blue scrubs under an old white lab coat, and she's slumped over the table on her elbows. Knowing Nina, I'm sure she'd much rather be delivering a baby than giving this presentation. She jiggles her foot up and down. Today she's changed her black clogs for sneakers that are so worn one toe curls up away from the sole, exposing her sock. There are old bloodstains on the leather.

The oncologist gets up for coffee, and when he returns to his place at the table the meeting begins. We all look intently at the handout that summarizes today's presentations, the patients' names indicated only by initials to ensure confidentiality. Those of us in the cheap seats share, looking over one another's shoulders.

Nina clears her throat and reads the first case:

"L.H. is a fifty-five-year-old Gravida four Para four, postmenopausal since age fifty-two, who initially presented to her private medical doctor with complaints of loss of appetite, increasing abdominal girth, and left lower quadrant pain. She denied other symptoms. On exam, patient was found to have a left-sided mass, and on pelvic ultrasound there was a normal retroverted uterus with a six-centimeter left complex adnexal mass. Patient was referred to her gynecologist.

"Past medical history is significant for gallstones and cholecystectomy in 1980. Appendectomy as a teenager.

"On June eighth, patient underwent total abdominal hysterectomy, bilateral salpingo-oophorectomy, and tumor debulking. A four-centimeter mass with multiple excrescences was noted on the omentum. The left ovary was adherent to the side wall. Uterus appeared free of disease, but the sigmoid colon had multiple nodules on the serosa which were removed. Palpable lymph nodes were removed. Liver and diaphragm were smooth. Pathology is pending."

Nina looks up and rustles her papers a bit. Someone gets up for more coffee. The language of medicine—so musical and complex, so encoded and distancing—is second nature to me. Here at

Tumor Board only as an observer, I decide it's my job to remember that there's a person behind the impermanent, melodious words.

"So," the oncologist says. "Nina."

Nina nods. "We debulked her as well as we could. There was a ton of fluid in her belly."

"Did you send it?"

"Yes. We sent a frozen but went ahead with the debulking before we got it back."

"We got pictures?" The oncologist looks over the table at the pathologist, who settles a cassette of slides into the projector, aims its tube of light at the screen pulled down over the blackboard, and stands, pulling out the tip of his pointer. The secretary jumps up to turn off the lights, and suddenly it's pitch-black. The projector clicks, and a photograph of L.H.'s left ovary appears on the screen.

The ovary, cut in half and pinned on an azure background, is red in some places and pink in others. In one spot the tumor has bubbled up, and there the screen is white. The pathologist walks up to the screen and taps the pointer against the tumor, making the screen waver.

"Here you can see gross tumor, and here"—he moves the pointer—"is the normal mucosa. Next."

One of the residents clicks the projector, and the second slide falls into place, the woman's uterus, right ovary, and fallopian tube against the same azure background. I'm struck by how *human* it is, yet we all sit here impassively, as if this once-alive organ had never been part of a woman who isn't here but always belonged to medicine, to us. Disengaging the specimen, the *thing,* from the living body is not easy to do. Even though I've seen slides like this many times before, studying the luminous flesh of the disembodied uterus makes me dizzy.

"You see this small area on the superior fundus? It turned out to be a fibroid. Next."

Again a click. The blank screen glistens, and then another slide appears.

"Here you have the field on higher power. You can see the prominent nucleoli. Notice the back-to-back cells, and here considerable vascular space invasion is evident."

The pathologist draws imaginary circles with his pointer. Next to me, a medical student has fallen asleep. Once in a while his head snaps back and he opens his eyes.

In the dark, the oncologist's voice is almost soothing. "Nina," he drones. "Tell us your guess on the histologic type."

She pauses a moment, trying to decide. "Well," she replies, "it could be serious cystadenocarcinoma."

The pathologist points. "There's significant lymphatic invasion over here." The pointer makes a dull sound against the screen, and the screen sways again, blurring L.H.'s ovarian cells.

I'm feeling a little nauseated, and I can't decide if it's the breakfast I ate too quickly or the thought of L.H., the fifty-five-year-old woman whose uterus and ovaries we're inspecting. She's probably at home right now waiting to hear from her doctor while we're here talking about what treatment might give her the best chance of survival. I conjure her in her kitchen getting a second cup of tea. This makes her so real to me, I can't help going on to fabricate her entire life. Other than the vague pain that stabs her along the healing surgical incision, she feels good. For once in her life, she's got it all together. Her daughter is doing well, graduated from Boston University last year on scholarships, and L.H. and her husband have made it through all these years in spite of money problems and one year during which she wondered what significance her life had, if any.

In the hospital, her doctor had looked serious when he had told her about the extent of her disease. Then he had sent her home "to recover," he'd said, and promised to call soon with plans for treatment. "A conference with specialists," he'd told her. "Get everyone's best opinion." Exactly what Emily and I said to Eleanor. But it's impossible for patients to imagine what really happens here, not only the impersonal, power-shifting arguments, but also the almost unbelievable effort that goes into defeating a patient's illness: the study, thought, and accumulated knowledge of this disparate group.

The lights-on secretary jumps up, and the room is ablaze again. Nina fidgets, her black hair shining. It's time for everyone to ask her questions, to grill her about this case. The oncology fellow from New York and the radiation oncologist and the surgeon lean forward in their chairs.

Before they can ask, Nina says, "Chemo and radiation are indicated."

The oncologist asks, "So what chemotherapy do you want to use?" and she answers, "Platinum," but she's unsure about what other agents are in vogue now, so her voice falters, giving the others their opportunity. Everyone talks at once. The doctors begin quoting articles and statistics, each man convinced of his own authority.

This is where I lose them. Until now I've been quite present, recognizing the large, irregular nuclei that randomly divide and crowd out the healthy cells, and the basement membrane that tries to protect the tissues but has been broken by tumor, and the small thin space that represents a lymph vessel with the small rosy fragment inside that means the tumor is already coursing through pellmell on its journey.

When statistics begin filling the air like torn scraps of paper, I find it harder to hold on to the image of L.H. If I let go of her now, she'll fall down and down into a murky place behind all the clinical words and facts, a chasm so deep she'll never be found. And Eleanor, whose case is next? I could never crumple Eleanor into a fistful of statistics.

I realize that now, like Lila, I'm the one engaged in magical thinking, as if I could change or direct a patient's future. If I envision her healed, she will be. If I suspect a more ominous outcome, I only have to shake my head and alter the plot, dispelling both the vision and the possibility. Perhaps this magical thinking connects in some way to poetry, the ability to suspend time and reality in order to enter more fully into the strange or the unknown, to live inside an idea or another's experience. Whatever its source, I like this pretending. It lets me relate viscerally to my patients, and it lets me, in some inexplicable way, participate in their care in a heightened, intuitive manner. It lets me fly yet keeps me grounded in this actual, corporal world.

The oncology fellow from New York is half standing, trying to get his "We published the only series on the combination of

four agents" into the air, and "In the British study more than half
the women lived 33.2 months after completing the third course"
comes from another oncologist. The facts pile up on the table. The
air is thick with them.

L.H. washes her cup, stands looking out the window. Around
me, the Tumor Board is arguing, one doctor's face lighting up and
then another's. The pathologist waves his hand and says, "We have
to move on to the next case, so let's come to some agreement."
The secretary, who will write the official letter to L.H.'s private doctor recommending treatment, readies her pen. The room quiets.
Then L.H. slips away, beyond the reach of imagination. I catch a
last glimpse of her in bed in a dim, closed room. Emily takes Nina's
place at the table. We lean forward again to follow the tiny black
words as she reads them out loud to the group of us:

"Case two. E.M. is a forty-nine-year-old Gravida four Para three
with no history of significant medical illness. She presented to the
clinic for an annual exam in March. She has a history of HPV but
denies prior abnormal Paps. Last Pap was five years ago and apparently normal. The Pap done in March returned 'ASCUS.' A Pap
done at a second visit returned 'Dysplasia, high grade, can't rule
out adenocarcinoma.' A colposcopy was done. The transformation
zone was seen, and there were mosaicism and white epithelium at
five and eight o'clock. Three biopsies were taken; two returned
'Carcinoma in situ, suggestive of microinvasion.' An endometrial
biopsy was negative, and the ECC was negative."

Emily looks up for a moment to make sure everyone is with
her.

The projector clicks. The slide of Eleanor's cervical cells looks
like a painting, swirls of maroon and blue that occasionally line up
into columns, here and there punctuated with scarlet dots.

The pathologist taps the screen with his pointer. "Right here,"
he says, "you see loss of normal cellular stratification and pleo-
morphism."

Another click. "Here it is in higher magnification. There's some
mitotic activity," and he taps the screen again, *tap tap tap.*

The screen goes blank, and the lights-on secretary jumps up

again. The doctors look at Emily, and the oncologist nods. "Yes?" he says.

"The next step is a cone biopsy. Because of the suggestion of microinvasion. We don't want to miss anything higher up."

"How old is she again?" a surgeon asks.

"Almost fifty."

"Well, she's not going to be having any more children, so you certainly don't need to worry about future cervical incompetence."

"Right," Emily says. "We'll plan to do a pretty generous cone. If that's negative, we can follow her with Paps."

"And if it's not negative?" a surgeon asks.

"We'll proceed to hysterectomy," Emily says.

"Right, a simple hysterectomy is probably all she'll need. She might be cured just with the cone."

The Tumor Board seems quite proud of itself, and Emily smiles at me. In the grand scheme of cancer, Eleanor's case is nothing, a little gnat, a pesky no-see-um buzzing around the room. We've gotten the word from the generals, and the word is that they're not worried.

Tumor Board is over, and the room empties. Nina goes up to Labor and Delivery, the medical students and residents hurry back to their rounds, the surgeons go to their surgeries, the oncologists to their bone marrow biopsies, and Emily and I head for the clinic.

Before I go, I invent Eleanor, sitting calmly near me in the row of folding chairs. I wink at her, and she grins at me. *Great news,* I say to her, *although brace yourself. There's a way to go to get there.* The vision begins to fade, and I reach out to clasp on to her. *Not so fast, Eleanor. I'm not about to let you get away.*

Sensuality, one of the loveliest attributes of the female body, is all around me in the clinic. Women come in smelling of soap and perfume. The Latinas arrive with their long, blue-black hair just washed; when they get up from the exam table, they leave a damp butterfly imprint on the paper. Asian women lift their shirts to reveal satiny cords tied around their bellies, talismans we cannot cut or remove for fear of releasing their souls. Patients from Brazil wear iridescent spandex tights and high heels that click up and down the hallway. When Pakistani women unfold their saris, the scent of cooking spices and sandalwood wafts into the air. Joanna, like our more prosperous patients, chooses perfume. Tonight, when she walks into my clinic out of the damp, end-of-summer evening air, she leaves a subtle, vaporous trail.

Evidence of sexuality, or what society deems to be sexual, abounds in the clinic as well: breasts, pubic hair, blood that's bright vermilion or black as ink, the moist mucosa that shows up pink and glistening under the light. There is also ample evidence of rebellion or abuse: tattoos on tender skin, a thin gold wire through the eyebrow or the clitoris, the swollen puff of a healing bruise. I see ecstatic newlyweds as well as women betrayed, newly diagnosed with a sexually transmitted disease. I see women in love with their sexual potential as well as women like Joanna, who find themselves drawing back, afraid. So many women are caught in the conflicts that arise when sensuality and sexuality collide.

What does it mean to be sexy, to be desirable? How does a woman's need for closeness, nurturing, safety, or risk influence her sexual behavior? How does sex serve as communication or as a substitute for communication? How does a woman learn to speak up and be clear about what she wants and doesn't want in a relationship? I think about these issues all the time.

Just as a poet develops a "voice"—an expression of her particular outlook or point of view that gives constancy and recognition to a body of work—every woman develops and hones her sexual voice over a lifetime. In the clinic, this voice is both actual and metaphoric. It's how a particular woman walks and talks, her attitude, her physical symptoms, the words she chooses to give shape to her fears and the experiences unique to her time. There are other voices, too, mine and the doctor's and the greater voice of society's customs and institutions. Often, all of us are talking at once.

As I open the door to room 2 and greet Joanna, who sits not on the exam table like a patient but on the straight-back chair in the corner like a friend dropped by for a chat, I realize that helping her, helping any woman, isn't always about what I've figured out and so can teach her. This evening, my role is to listen, not judging what Joanna might reveal but supporting her as she strives to define her self. Listening might be all I can do to help her find her safe place.

"Hi, Joanna," I say, extending my hand to her. "It's good to see you again." When I'd phoned weeks ago to say that her test results showed no syphilis, no hepatitis, no chlamydia or gonorrhea from her "one-night stand," she was relieved. But when I asked if she had scheduled an appointment with one of the therapists, she'd said no, she hadn't had time. Besides, she was *sure* her pelvic pain was caused by something physical. She'd gone on to tell me she felt so angry at David she could hardly stand it, but she didn't know why. He was being kind and understanding. She was being a bitch.

Then she'd never kept the follow-up appointment we'd made

to discuss her HIV test and the status of her pain, when I'd been so sure she would honor that agreement. "She blew you off," my assistant had said. Patient's prerogative, I replied. Joanna knew she'd hear from me if there was a problem. I thought about calling her again but, still cautious about pushing too hard, talked myself out of it. If she wanted to, she'd return. It wouldn't be the first time a woman simply disappeared, the outcome of her symptoms forever unknown to me.

"Hi," Joanna says. A thin eggshell blue scarf is knotted around her throat.

I sit down and tell her that the HIV screen was negative.

"Thank God," she says, and her shoulders sag. "I thought you'd call me if it wasn't, but it's good to hear for sure."

"It would be best if you had another test in a few months," I add. "There's a window of time after exposure before a test converts to positive. So repeating the test is very important."

Joanna nods. Then there are a few seconds of silence. We both seem unsure of how to resume our dialogue.

"You remember that swelling I told you about?" she says. "I notice that now the other side is swollen too."

Ah. Joanna has returned to bring me proof. There *is* something structurally wrong with her body. She can point to the swelling and think, here it is. Now, if only I could locate the offending spot and take it out. A momentary glitch in Joanna's anatomy, a foreign body that I might discover and name, and so banish.

One day a thirty-year-old woman came into the clinic in a panic. She'd found, she said, a lump on the outside of her vagina. When I examined her, I was astonished to find that she meant her clitoris, that nub of sensitive tissue that hides in the labial folds above the vagina. Could I believe that a woman was so ignorant of her own body? Yes, yet often there is more to such a seemingly naïve question. Maybe such an approach is the only way a woman can begin to ask for help. What would happen if a woman like that took her question to a caregiver who laughed, gave a brief explanation, then walked away? On a hunch, I asked her about her relationships. She was married and had two children. I asked her about abuse. Yes, her father had "been mean" to her in childhood, and her husband, when he was angry or drunk, shoved and shook her in the same way. Now he was hitting her, too, belittling her in front of their children. She'd never enjoyed sex, ever. Unlike Joanna, that patient and I talked openly, and she asked for help. I called the women's center, which sent someone right over. My patient and her children fled to a shelter.

Joanna looks around the room, and I wonder if she's trying to figure out who was here before her. An infected woman? A woman with AIDS? A woman who was once abused?

I decide to take the initiative.

"Joanna, I'm not sure what's going on with your pain, but as you know, I think it might have an emotional component, not just something in your head but some specific cause. That's why I suggested therapy. I'm concerned that you didn't make an appointment."

"What kind of emotional component?" Joanna asks.

"Sometimes, as we've been talking, I've sensed there were other things on your mind, things that might be difficult to talk about but would have some connection to the pelvic pain. Emotional issues often reveal themselves through physical symptoms."

Joanna crosses and uncrosses her legs. She begins to slouch, to get comfortable, and then her shoulders stiffen, as if an unseen adult has poked her, reminding her to sit up straight.

"I've known David for a long time. I'm in love with him," she says. "Other than *my* not wanting to have sex, there's nothing wrong with our relationship."

She has decided to talk about David and their perfect, but asexual, partnership, so I go along.

"How did you and David meet?"

"We went to the same college, but we didn't really date until our senior year. Actually, I was the one who probably changed our relationship from friendship to something more... serious, I guess. He says he fell in love with me right away, that he'd loved me all the time we were friends but was afraid to say anything. We went out for that whole year, but then I went to Italy for graduate studies and he stayed in school in Ohio."

Joanna, I notice, is freely revealing personal, emotional infor-

mation to me. Before, her words were measured, more cautiously
dispensed. Maybe she knows me well enough now and is more at
ease. Maybe the weeks in between our visits have given her time to
think, time to listen to the daydreams and nightmares that might
hint at her internal turmoil. Whatever the reason, I'm grateful. I
act as if we've been talking this easily all along.

"Did you continue your relationship with David while you
were away?"

"Sort of. I didn't date anyone else, and he came to Italy to visit
me a few times. It was there that I knew that I loved him, too. It
surprised me."

"Falling in love with him surprised you?"

"I'd always felt really close to him, you know, like best friends.
But when we were in Italy together he seemed . . . I don't know, so
much *like* me. He *understood* me. When he went back to Ohio, all
I could think about was how much I wanted to be with him."

"Then, when you got home to Ohio?"

"I decided not to move in with him, even if my parents *might*
have eventually adjusted. I sort of wanted to save living together
for marriage, you know? A little old-fashioned."

"Not at all," I say. "As you were growing up, did your parents
give you any indication of how they felt about sex? It sounds like
they might have been pretty strict."

Joanna laughs, but the snapshot she presents of her family is
bleak: "My mother handed me a book on menstruation, and once I
began dating, every time someone came to pick me up they'd say,
'If you ever get pregnant, you can just plan on moving out of here.'
I never saw my parents kiss or hug."

I nod. "I think I was handed that same book."

Joanna touches the scarf around her neck. I let a moment go
by. No more than five seconds.

"Do you feel any guilt now about being with David?"

She hesitates. Then she continues, and, carefully, I follow along.

"I don't think so. I mean, I *am* a grown woman. I think, too,
that when my mother died I felt more . . . more independent, I suppose. Actually, one of the main reasons I didn't move in with David

right away was my career. It was important to me, you understand. But I always knew I'd marry him eventually."

"What kind of work does he do?"

"He's a chemist." She says this with a little twitch of her nose. "He's the scientist, I'm the artist."

"So what attracts you to him?"

She seems thrown by this question, as if she'd never thought about it before.

"Well, he's very kind. He's smart and likes to do a lot of things I enjoy, travel and hiking. I know he'd make a wonderful father. He makes me feel happy. I can't imagine not being with him." She pauses, looks down, smoothes her hair. "Can I ask you a question?"

"Of course," I say. *Of course. Keep going, Joanna.*

"What does 'frigid' mean?" she says.

"Not much," I answer. "I think that label is applied to any woman who doesn't want to have sex when someone else wants her to. But that has nothing to do with the separate issue of a woman's degree of sexual response. If a man can't sustain an erection, no one calls him frigid."

"Well, sex with David has always been . . . OK. I mean, it's not him. There's something wrong with *me*."

"Was sex ever enjoyable for you, Joanna, with any other partners?"

She hesitates. "No, it's always been about the same. It seemed better with David in the beginning."

I jump off a high platform, hoping there's a safety net. "Do you experience orgasm? Any way at all? Through masturbation, by your partner stimulating your clitoris, or by vaginal penetration?"

"I don't masturbate." She makes a face. "Sometimes I have an orgasm if David stimulates me. But it takes so long I usually just pretend. That's why I wonder if I'm frigid. I have this friend who always tells me how wonderful sex is, how she has all these multiple orgasms."

"The majority of women require direct clitoral stimulation in order to reach orgasm. In fact, it's very common for women *not* to achieve orgasm vaginally, although some do. I also have patients who have never experienced orgasm at all. Sex takes practice and a good deal of talking. It takes a lot of trust as well."

"David has tried, but I don't really like to talk about sex."

Joanna, I see, has decided to ignore the word "trust." Perhaps when she lived alone in New York, when she could lose herself in her art and ignore her body, she had a different voice. Now, it seems, she has given up her voice completely. More likely, I think, she was silenced very early and has never had a voice at all.

"In Italy, David and I couldn't wait to be together. We'd get into a room and begin tearing our clothes off."

"Tell me about Italy."

"Oh, it was wonderful. I sketched in the museums all day, and when I got home David was there, waiting for me. I'd paint, we'd go out to dinner and then for a long walk. I felt like a whole person."

"And now?"

"Now I'm always annoyed. When he tries to hug me when I'm about to make dinner or when he gives me those signals that mean he wants to have sex. Sometimes I wonder if he wants it to be like it used to, when we'd tear off our clothes and fall on the floor."

"Have you ever asked him?"

Joanna gestures, an opening of her hand. "No, I suppose I haven't."

"When everything is new, you don't demand as much from a relationship," I say. "It's flattering to think 'He loves me so much he can't wait to be with me,' but over time successful lovemaking requires careful planning more than spontaneity. Lots of talking and stimulation. The permission to be yourself. Too many of us are conditioned by movies and TV to believe that good relationships have to be forever urgent and sexually charged."

Once I had a patient whose partner had walked out, complaining he no longer found her exciting. She had looked at me with the wry humor that eventually comes to survivors and said, "Wouldn't you like to get the person who invented the Ken and Barbie myth?"

"Anyway," Joanna continues, "I was a different person in Italy. I can remember what it was like, but I can't recapture that feeling."

"So you don't feel like a whole person anymore."

She looks at me, and I see that behind her glasses, her eyes are olive brown. "Not really. I feel pressured and out of place."

"Since you moved in with David?"

"Yeah," she says. "Maybe before that, too."

"Have you told David that you feel pressured? That you'd rather not have sex those times when he wants to and you don't?"

Joanna looks down at the floor. She looks back at me.

"Usually I go along with it," she says. "I don't want to hurt him." Then she adds, "It's easier than trying to get into all the excuses."

I pause a moment, wondering if Joanna hears her own words. "Joanna," I say. "Tell me about the first time you and David had sex. How was it decided that you would begin having sex? And who decided? Do you remember?"

She thinks a moment. "Nobody really decided. We were friends for so long. I guess it was me who made the first move. One night after we'd been out with a bunch of friends, I kissed David goodnight, like I always did. But this time I kept kissing him. The next night he asked me what I wanted, and I told him I wanted him. I thought that's what he would want me to say."

"Is that what *you* wanted to say?"

"I didn't think about it. The words just came out."

Like the affair just happened. Like the pain just started.

"Sometimes now I'm afraid that if I hug David, he'll think I want to have sex, when all I want is a hug."

She turns away. When she and David make love, I wonder if she just lies there as she did during her pelvic exam, vacant-eyed and tolerant. I wonder which woman Joanna really is—the independent student in Italy who lugged her easel and paints from hilltop to grotto or the agreeable Joanna who reluctantly submits. Maybe she's both.

"So in the early part of your relationship you felt more . . ."

"Free."

Joanna straightens her shoulders and stretches her legs. I sense it's time to back off and try going down another path. I'm hoping that by simply asking questions, I will get Joanna to think about some issues that we women often don't address when considering our relationships and how we've come to be in them, or our problems and how they may have evolved.

I ask if her dad remarried after her mother died. He never dated anyone, Joanna says. Her mother was only fifty-one when she was killed in a car accident.

"I don't think he ever got over it," she says.

"How about you?" I ask. "How are you doing?"

She shrugs. Her cheeks become deep pink and her eyes fill, silvery crescents mirrored in the rim of each lower lid. "It was pretty tough," she says. "Still is."

I ask if anything about her parents' relationship gives her any insight into her own relationship patterns, and Joanna smirks.

"My mother was sort of a free spirit. I wanted to be like her, but I'm more like my dad. Serious, the brooding temperament. Before my mother died, she'd begun sort of living her own life, doing her own thing if he didn't want to go along."

"How about you and David? Do you make a point of spending time together, or do you tend to drift into separate activities?"

She's quiet for a moment. "It seems like the only time we get together now is in bed. And that certainly isn't great."

I feel the isolation in her words physically, cold as a handful of ice shards.

"Did you have any other role models for relationships, growing up? Like grandparents or aunts and uncles? Family friends?"

Joanna shifts around in her chair and grips the edges of the seat with her hands, all of a sudden restless. "Not really."

She looks around as if searching for a fork in the road that will turn the conversation in another direction.

"Anyway, sometimes I think David would be better off without me."

"Do you want to break up with him?"

"Oh no," she says, shocked. "I love David. And I have no desire to get back into the dating scene. I hear my friends talk about it all the time."

I hear the residents talk a lot about dating too. Two of them are married, and the others are looking. Not desperate, but keeping their eyes open. One resident tried computer dating. She e-mailed a man for weeks. Eventually, they met for coffee on neutral ground. They liked each other and ventured into a cautious series of dates. At first, things seemed to be going well. When I asked how her love life was, she'd smile and say, "Not so bad!" A month later I asked again, and she said it was over. "He wasn't my type," she said. "I decided it was better just to cut it off. Why waste his time or mine?"

"What do your friends say?" I ask Joanna.

"That it's horrible and there's too much to think about."

"What would be some of your concerns?"

"What if I got into another relationship and it didn't work out? Then I'd have to start all over again at square one. Or what if I fell in love with someone and he wasn't ready? I want to have kids, not right away, but what if I never met anyone and then I was too old? Educational level is important to me too. And my own career, what *I* want to do. Lots of things are important. You have to be so perfect today. God, the thought of getting naked in front of a new man terrifies me."

Joanna's questions and worries cascade out, all of them valid— many of them, I realize, different issues than my friends and I faced. We didn't agonize so much over the right person, the right goals, and the right time. Maybe we should have. Marriage and children were a given, and several of my friends married their high school sweethearts right after graduation. Now we justify our lack of vigilance by saying we were more willing to compromise than the young people today. Then again, our divorce rate was 50 percent. No wonder our children are scared. In the clinic I see both ends of the spectrum, women who fall into and out of relationships and pregnancies with little self-awareness and women who might analyze a relationship to death.

Outside the door, I hear voices, my assistant requesting, "Could you bring your urine specimen back into room four?" and then the quiet reply of my next patient. Joanna hears this as well. We both sit a moment, just looking at each other. We've been talking for an hour, a rare luxury even in the evening clinic.

"So," I say.

This is what I've been waiting for, through all of Joanna's visits:

a way in, the tiniest of handholds. And now it's time for our conversation to end. Nevertheless, I know how these things work. Someone says something or asks a question, and that sets a chain of thought and memory into motion. It may be her reflection, not our talking, that leads Joanna to revelation.

Before we walk out into the hallway, I turn to her.

"Joanna, it seems as if you have a lot to discuss with a therapist. I understand how difficult it would be to start talking to someone new. But a therapist will be better able to help you than I am." Again I write the names of the three therapists I initially suggested and hand the list to Joanna. "This doesn't mean I won't continue to see you, too. I'm here for you anytime. Will you keep in touch?"

It must be lonely for Joanna, I think, having all these things to talk about and no one to talk to.

"Yes," she says. "I'll keep in touch."

I detain her a moment, just the pressure of my hand on her arm. "Could I give you two exercises to try at home?"

"Sure," she answers.

"The first is to make a list of words, just verbs and nouns, that you'd use to describe who you are. Write them down quickly, as many as you can. Bring the list in with you next time. The second exercise might be more difficult."

"Shoot," she says.

"When David wants to make love and you don't, tell him. If you can't say no when you don't feel like having sex, nothing will ever change."

Chapter 21

It's late September. Lila, now twenty-seven weeks pregnant, has missed several appointments. The phone number she gave me for Charles's mother's apartment is out of service, and a registered letter sent to the apartment address was returned unclaimed.

"How much can you do?" one of the nurses asked. "Don't patients have any responsibility for themselves?"

I called the visiting nurse, Rita, and asked if she would look for Lila at the last address she had given us, 45 Berry Road, apartment 4B.

At 45 Berry Road, Rita said, Charles's mother came to the door. A small, heavy woman, she shrugged her shoulders and whisked her hands together as if to say "Well rid of them."

She said that Lila and Charles had moved out weeks ago but not to ask her where they were: "I don't know, and I don't much care."

Then Rita tried Lila's old apartment, but the young girl living there said she had no idea who Lila was. Besides, the girl was suspicious. *What do you want to know for anyway?*

Rita asked around town, at the shelter and at the women's center, but no one knew Lila. A few girls knew Charles but hadn't seen him in months. They laughed. *Found someone to clip his wings, did he?*

In the back room, Nina and Emily and I look at each other. Now what? We make a big note on Lila's chart: "At next visit, ask Lila where she's living." What's going on? It isn't like Lila to avoid prenatal care. Before this, she'd made it to every appointment. Is she drugging? Is she in trouble?

"She's not the only one I have to keep track of, you know." Rita sheds her raincoat, shaking water and leaves off her hair, a mass of gray kinks and curls. "Poodle hair," she calls it. Rita has come to the clinic for our weekly high-risk conference, a multidisciplinary meeting of doctors, residents, nurses, the social worker, the visiting nurse, and one of the drug rehab counselors. We get together to talk about managing our problem patients, including the pregnant teenagers. The cafeteria supplies a tray of bagels and fruit and a pot of strong coffee to help us sort through the morass of difficulties our patients face.

Rita is correct. Lila is only one problem in a truckload of problems. One lost pregnant fifteen-year-old whose dilemmas, big as they are, aren't as great as they might be. Rita, who goes daily into the city and the suburbs armed with her black bag and her blue visiting nurse uniform, sees a lot worse. She's the undisputed horror story queen.

Rita always says there's something about our patients' lives that makes our troubles seem small. Take Maria, for example, one of our patients who lived in the worst apartment complex in the city. She'd been pregnant not too long ago, three years maybe. After her son was born, she didn't have transportation into the clinic for her six-week postpartum check, and besides, she'd recently separated from an abusive husband and was afraid to go out. He'd beaten her during the pregnancy, and now he was stalking her, calling and pleading, saying he loved her and couldn't live without her. Then, an hour later, he'd appear at her door, pounding and screaming that she had no right to keep him from his family. Rita started visiting Maria and her son, Michael, every week, partly to check on how Maria was recovering from her pregnancy, partly to make sure she was safe. Rita told us how she had to wend her way through the discarded needles and plastic bags left in the parking lot, and how she'd keep her eyes down to avoid the men who lounged at noon against the gates and stared at her. Maria would peer out the window like an anxious mother, watching Rita until she was in the hallway and out of jeopardy.

Maria had a restraining order against her husband, but that didn't seem to deter him. "Go ahead, call someone and report me," he'd shout from the parking lot. Then he'd throw garbage at her window. Wet sacks filled with half-eaten sandwiches would thud against the glass. Empty beer cans *ting*ed against the siding and bounced on the cement. "You bitch, you can't keep me from my son," he'd shout as all the women in the complex double-locked their doors. He filed a petition requesting sole custody, claiming that he was better able to support and raise his son. Maria, of course, didn't have money to fight back. She was supposed to return to work but didn't dare. Where, she asked, could she find a safe place to leave Michael? Anyway, before she was pregnant, she'd once tried to save money to leave her husband. When he'd found out, he'd punched her until her eyes closed and her cheek puffed up purple and squishy as a rotting plum. He began waiting for her at work, hassling her coworkers. "Don't you know she drinks?" he'd ask them. "Did you know she sees other men?" Maria became just another invisible woman unable to escape.

One Wednesday, Rita was sitting in the kitchen with Maria and nine-week-old Michael when someone started kicking the apartment door. Rita said Maria's face blanched and a fine sweat broke out on her upper lip. She handed her baby to Rita and propped a chair under the doorknob.

"Go away!" Maria yelled. "I've got the nurse here. You just go away and leave me alone." There was a moment of silence, then Rita heard a man's voice.

"OK. I'm sorry I bothered you." Maria's husband waited another minute, a slow, quiet space of time; then he went down the hall, his metallic footfall clanging softer and softer. For a moment, Rita thought, "He sounded polite"; his composed voice almost erased the memory of his brisk pounding. But when Rita went down the stairs after her visit, she found Maria's husband leaning against the railing, waiting.

"Hello," he said, moving out in front of her and grinning. His

face was tan and his cheeks were chapped, as if he did outdoor
work. His black hair was cut close and slicked straight back. He
smelled of aftershave, Rita noticed. His nose was short, pug, and
when he smiled, his teeth were small, even. There was something
about him, Rita told us later. He was almost charming.

"I hope I didn't scare you," he said, bending a little at the waist
and smiling again. "I just wanted to talk to you. I'm really worried
about Maria and the baby."

Rita stopped and clutched her nurse's bag in front of her with
both hands. She didn't say anything, but she didn't walk away, either. She could have pushed her way past him. "Get the hell out of
my way," she might have said.

"My Mike's quite a boy, isn't he? But I think Maria needs our
help."

Our help. This made her curious. And, in spite of all she knew,
it made Rita his accomplice.

Rita hesitated. Then she asked, "Why is that?"

He made a funny half bow, half shuffle that made him seem
childlike and ungainly.

"Well," he continued, "she's worked herself up so much I'm
worried that she's not thinking clearly. I worry about Mike. I mean,
what do you think? You're a professional. You just saw them. I'd
trust your judgment any day. Do you think she's depressed or
what? Can she take care of Mikey OK?"

"Mike looked perfectly well cared for," Rita said. In spite of
herself, she added, "He's adorable." Then she wished she could take
back her words.

"Looks like me," Maria's husband said, turning his profile to
Rita. "See my big old nose?" He laughed, and his cheeks got ruddier
and his hair seemed blacker and his eyes sparkled. *Handsome,* Rita
thought.

"By the way," he said. "Did Maria ever tell you my name?"

Rita thought a moment. She must have. Or did Maria never
mention his name, only how horrible he was? Maybe there was
something to his side of this after all. She actually thought this, she
told us, even though she had seen the bruises on Maria's body with
her own eyes.

"No," Rita said. "I don't remember if she ever mentioned your name."

"Billy," he said and held out his hand. It was square and rough. When Rita placed her hand in his, it was warm. He closed his fingers around hers a moment too long. It felt, she realized afterward, almost sexual.

"Billy," she repeated. "Well, I have to get going now. More patients to see." She shuffled her bag.

"Hey, let me carry that for you," he said and took the bag from her before she had time to clutch it closer. For a second she was afraid. She didn't carry anything in the bag anyone might want, no needles or drugs, just bandages, thermometers, a few diapers, and some tape. But when Billy walked out of the hallway into the daylight, gallantly holding the door for her, she felt silly. Obviously he didn't mean her any harm. She walked to her car and he followed; then he waited while she opened the door. He handed her the bag and stepped aside.

"Nice to meet you," he said. "Maybe we'll meet again."

As Rita drove away, she looked up at Maria's window. She saw a small face peering out from behind the greasy glass, the shadow of a woman watching them.

The next day, Rita got two phone calls. The first was from Maria. She sounded frantic and she spoke so fast Rita had to tell her, "Slow down."

"You may think he's nice, but he's a monster," Maria had said. "How could you talk to him? You're supposed to be helping *me!*"

Rita reassured her. Off the phone, she minimized Maria's fears. She wondered if Maria *was* a bit out of control. The next call Rita got that day was from Billy.

"Listen," he said, "I'm down here at the apartment. I just went over to the store and picked up a few things for Maria and the baby. You know, they've had it rough without my being there, and anyway formula was on sale. I figured I'd get a case for them, why not? Hey, I ended up getting two. So I wonder if you'd give me a hand and deliver the stuff to Maria?"

Rita must have gotten a funny look on her face, because one of the nurses mouthed, "What?" Rita shook her head. *Nothing.* Then she'd agreed to meet Billy and take the formula and groceries up to Maria for him. Rita told herself she was making a big deal out of nothing. The guy just wanted to help his own family.

She drove over and parked in the only open space near the complex. She could see Billy sitting on the run-down swing set that stood at one side of the lot on a small grassy patch. His legs were so long he just rocked himself back and forth on his heels, singing the rhythm to himself. When he saw Rita get out of her car, he jumped off, and the swing flipped up and started jittering on the chain. He reached her in a few strides.

"Thanks so much. It's really great, you going out like this for me and all."

"I'll just take the things upstairs if you show me where they are," Rita said. She told us later that her heart started to pound and she thought she should get into the car right then and call the police. She didn't know why she felt that way—the quiet voice inside, maybe. But she didn't listen.

"Oh, I put all the stuff in the hallway already. But you can't carry it. Come on, you're a little thing."

"Really, I'll get it."

"Come on, don't tell me you're one of those women who won't let a guy help her? I wouldn't have figured you for that type."

He paused a second and then smiled at her. Rita said she felt trapped.

"I'm not any type of woman, but I know that Maria has a restraining order against you. If you go up to the apartment, she'll call the police."

"Lighten up. She's not gonna call anybody. I'll carry the stuff up and leave it in front of the door. Then I'll go. Promise." He opened his hands, palms up. He smiled, his teeth as white as his pressed shirt. "Poof, like that. I'll be gone."

He took Rita's elbow and directed her up the entranceway stairs, then to the landing at the bottom of the two metal flights that led up to Maria's door. Rita thought about screaming, but she didn't. She thought about shoving her heavy bag smack into his face and then running, but she didn't.

"Where are the groceries?" Rita said, looking around.

"Oops, forgot. I took 'em up already. I got tired of waiting for you. They're sitting right outside Maria's door. So let's walk up and you knock and tell Maria it's OK for her to open up."

"It's not OK. I can't tell her that it is."

Billy hesitated and looked at her. "I thought you had to be smart to be a nurse. If you're smart, you'll tell her to open the door."

He gripped Rita's arm, and she was too frightened to pull away. They walked upstairs in silence. But once they were outside Maria's door, Rita shouted, "Maria! Call the police! Somebody, call the police!"

What happened next happened fast: "All I know is that he yelled something about her not calling the cops or he'd kill her, and then Maria opened the door a crack. He got in that door in a second and slammed it in my face."

Rita stood in the hallway immobilized for several seconds. She didn't hear any sound from inside the apartment. It took her another moment to realize that she was the one who had to call the police, and quickly. She knew that when women leave abusive partners, they often *increase* their risk. There's something about the actual act of separation that escalates the violence. Rita knew this, yet somehow she'd been taken in.

She threw her bag on the floor and pawed through it to find her cell phone. She dialed 911 and reported domestic violence. She told the policewoman on the line to get someone over there fast because she thought Billy might kill Maria. It took two officers a lifetime to arrive.

"Police! Open the door!" they shouted. Rita moved out of their way and froze.

"Police!" they bellowed, banging the door, rattling it almost off its frame. "Open up!"

"For God's sake, Maria! Open the door!" Rita said. She heard Mikey begin to cry, a piercing wail. Then Billy opened the door and stood with his hands on his hips, grinning. "What's the problem, officer? You-all are making a lot of noise. You woke my son up." Maria appeared behind him. She wore her robe and held Mikey. Both of their faces were blotchy and slick with tears.

"Don't look at me. I didn't do anything," Billy said.

The police pushed into the apartment, their navy uniforms studded with shiny buttons, their thick leather belts creaking as they walked.

"What's going on here?" one of the cops said.

"I'm the baby's father. I came to deliver some food and formula. Taking care of the family, you know? You got kids, officer?"

Rita stood perfectly still on the landing. "Maria has a restraining order against her husband," she said. "He's been abusive in the past."

The police looked at Maria. "Did he hurt you, ma'am?"

Maria whispered, "No."

Billy shook his head. "Come on, man. I told you. I was just bringing them some food." He indicated the bags of groceries on Maria's table. "That's all I wanted. And to see my son. Now I'm out of here." He walked closer to Maria and she recoiled, ducking her face behind the bulk of Michael's blanket. Billy curled his lip. He kissed Maria as she turned away in disgust; then he bent over and kissed the baby's cheek.

One cop escorted Billy, and the other stayed to complete some paperwork with Maria. Rita, her heart thudding, clambered down the two flights of narrow, litter-strewn stairs, hurried past the men still lounging by the gate, past the needles and the bags and the three-year-olds playing on the slide, past the mothers who were watching them, past the police cruiser that sat with its light going around and around, past the puddles of oily water pooled by the curb, past the junked cars that took up parking spaces, past the green plastic bags of garbage that stank to high heaven, finally to her own Ford hatchback with one ding on the right front fender. Her hands shook so much she could hardly get the key in.

––––––––––––––––

We all knew how it had ended. None of us ever saw Billy again. Apparently, we thought, he'd finally given up and moved on. Maria was granted a divorce, and after several months the courts allowed Billy to see Michael under third-party supervision. We saw Maria a couple of times in the clinic, and she seemed happy, back on track. Rita continued to visit her once in a while at home. When Michael was about a year and a half old, Maria found a new boyfriend.

One day, Rita came into work and told us that Billy had just broken into Maria's apartment in a fit of rage and stabbed her to death. We couldn't believe it. Anyone who has worked in health care for a while has seen and heard a lot. Even here in our suburban clinic, miles away from a typical high-crime area, evidence of tragedy and oppression is commonplace. Still, nothing ever prepares us for the unexpected horrors. "Why?" we asked each other when Rita told us this story. "Why?"

We know the statistics by heart, yet they don't seem possible or real until something like this happens, a disaster that comes too close, like a woman who walks past us on the sidewalk and catches our eye, her face holding the memory of a close call. To everyone else reading the newspaper that day, Maria was an anonymous woman who became another victim of domestic violence—something that happens to someone else, to women who are not like us, women who are poor, on welfare, of color, or "asking for it." But I *knew* Maria. I'd joked with her and felt Michael squirming beneath her belly when I'd measured the long nine months of her pregnancy. I'd worried when Rita had told us about Billy, and I remembered Maria's shy manner and how she liked to bring us brownies plump with raisins and chocolate chips because she knew we liked them that way. We all remembered calling the women's shelter for her. We remembered Billy lurking in the waiting room. We remembered talking in high-risk conference about how women are more likely to be battered during pregnancy, how women on welfare are more likely to be victims of abuse, and how there is plenty of "suburban" violence as well. It's just better hidden. We had our stories, too, we middle-class professionals. How, while in the midst of a divorce or a custody battle or in the heat of an argument, some of us had had our own close calls. The sarcastic remark that cut like a knife. The threatening phone message at work. *Don't come home. I'm waiting.* The shove that had become a punch.

Rita said she was glad for one thing: When the police initially had taken Billy away, Rita had returned the next day and apologized to Maria. She said she'd let Billy sucker her in when she should have known better. She said she'd learned something she would never forget. Maria was the victim. She was sorry for letting her allegiance to Maria slip, even for a moment. Rita stood up and walked over, put her hand on Maria's shoulder. The bones under her sweater were edgy and moved with quick, unsure movements. "I'm so sorry," Rita had said.

———————————

High-risk conference usually lasts about an hour. Afterward, some of us hang around to clear the table and hide the leftover bagels for the next day. Rita stays with us, not eager to go out into the chilly rain again. She looks tired. Like all of us, she has problems of her own. She gets out her notebook and lines up tomorrow's route: "Stop at the halfway house, check on Jamie. Bring food to Madeleine. Check the women's shelters again for Lila."

Chapter 22

"Hey," Loretta says. She has a stethoscope around her neck and wears a cranberry print smock over a white skirt. Pink and blue baby beads tied to the stethoscope spell out her name.

"Yeah, hey," says Renée, and the two of them press closer to Marvin's Isolette.

I'm here as Renée's chaperone, although I could have told her that I was too busy and that someone from Detox would have to escort her. I guess I want to see her succeed. I remember that streak of cynicism that stirred within me, years ago, when I asked myself how I could go on believing any patient after I had been so fooled by Renée. She was the one who shook my foundation of trust. Now I want to give her a chance to be, instead, one of the many patients who gives me the strength to keep listening.

Loretta takes Renée by the shoulders, turns her so they're face-to-face. Renée's all dressed up today, though she still wears the same faded pull-on slippers. Her lips are deep red with a dash of lipstick. She has a crescent of blue smudged above each eye.

Loretta asks Renée to unbutton her blouse.

"This is how you kangaroo a baby," Loretta says. "You'll hold Marvin's bare body against your skin. He will feel your breathing and hear your heartbeat, and this helps him to regulate his own. It teaches him to breathe. In and out. In and out."

She helps as Renée fumbles with her buttons.

"Take it easy," Loretta says. "No hurry."

Renée's fingers shake. Loretta gives her a quick hug and whispers something in her ear that I can't hear. Renée laughs. "Kangaroo you, too," she says.

Loretta drags the rocking chair from across the room and moves it close to Marvin's Isolette. She props up the lid and lifts Marv out. Wrapped tight in his flannel blanket, he's a small bundle, a leg of lamb tied in butcher paper, a smooth loaf of bread. Loretta unwinds the tubes and catheters that stitch themselves around the baby.

"Oh, man," Renée says. "I really gotta hold him?"

Loretta doesn't speak, just continues to peel away Marvin's layers until he's bare except for a white rumpled preemie diaper that still looks too big and the gauze padding that protects his intravenous lines.

"Maybe I better not," says Renée. "You know, maybe it'd be better if I didn't. I'm a little shaky today, you know?"

"You'll do fine," Loretta says. "You're his mother, and you'll hold him just fine."

"I better not drop him," Renée says.

Loretta motions Renée into the rocking chair, and she sits, her blouse open, her skin dull and velvety. Loretta lifts Marvin. She swings him down, and for a moment his arms and legs startle and he flies. When his body touches Renée's chest, he clings instinctively, a baby clutching his mother's warmth, a matter of life and death.

Renée is so afraid she quivers. Loretta massages her arms, her shoulders.

"Relax," she says. "Relax your whole body. He'll feel you relax, and he'll relax too. Shhhhhh," she says. "Shhhhhh."

Renée dips her chin, trying to control her trembling, and she takes big deep breaths. Loretta just stands there, as if she has no doubt in the world that Renée can do this simple, impossible task.

I try hard to watch what's happening here. I try to learn something about being kind.

Renée begins to rock, pushing herself back and forth with the tip of her slipper, and the chair goes *crik-crik, crik-crik.* Her back yields, then her arms, then she rests her elbow on the chair's arm and snuggles her baby closer. It occurs to me that her other children were taken away immediately after birth; this may be the first time she's ever held or rocked a child. Until now, she couldn't even have imagined what this was like. No wonder she was resentful, careless about her pregnancy, having been denied the pleasure of her other three babies' bodies against her breast.

Marvin responds. He burrows his floppy head into her, and his skin steams and sticks to hers, vaporizing her perfume and his lotion. A sweet smell rises in the air around them. His hair is curly and the color of black wine, much darker than her flesh. His rheumy eyes are open, his head back, his mouth dry and empty and round, and he watches her with the wisdom of an ancient, wizened man, as if he knows everything already and loves her anyway.

She rocks and hums, cradling Marvin's naked scrawny body against her bare skin. Loretta and I move away into the shadows. Renée rocks and murmurs. Marvin sleeps, swaying on that suspension bridge between the world he came from and the one he's in now.

When Loretta finally says it's time to put Marvin back in his house, I see one tear on Renée's cheek, but she quickly wipes it away. I wish the nurses who doubted Renée's intentions could see what I see: a woman who loves her child, a mother whose sorrow at leaving him is genuine.

"Come back tomorrow, and we'll do this again," Loretta says.

Renée gives Marvin a long look. "See ya tomorrow, Marv," she says.

I walk with her out to the elevator on our way back to Detox. We're quiet until the elevator arrives on seven and she has to get out, back to her group meetings and her bitter-tasting methadone in a paper cup and her stark room with its metal bed and single dresser.

"So, wow," Renée says and smiles at me as if she'd just come from a party.

Chapter 23

The uterus, if you could peer into the body to see it, looks like a pink, smooth pear. Pluck the green leaf, remove the stem, and imagine the pear turned upside down. The rounded end of the pear is the body of the uterus, smooth and firm. The narrow neck of the pear is the cervix, the only part of the uterus that protrudes into the vagina where it can be seen and touched, the part of Eleanor's body that has gone awry, turning itself, cell by cancerous cell, against her.

The small hole where the stem was plucked out is the cervical os, from the Latin word for "mouth," the opening of the passageway that leads through the cervix into the uterine cavity. This endocervical canal might be thought of as a path and the os as the doorway; menstrual blood is propelled from the uterine cavity down the canal to the external os, where it escapes into the vagina. Sperm swim from the vagina into the external os and through the endocervical canal. Reaching the end of the canal, they pass through the internal os into the uterus and on to the fallopian tubes in search of a woman's ovum. If sperm and egg meet, they lock together and migrate back to the uterine cavity, dividing as they go. The ensuing pregnancy is complete when the baby is pushed by rhythmic uterine contractions out through the dilated cervix.

The uterus sits low in a woman's body, tucked between the bladder in front and the rectum in back. This is why a woman must drink water to expand her bladder before an ultrasound; the bladder becomes a window through which the uterus can be seen. In an instinctive desire to soothe her uterus, a woman experiencing menstrual cramps massages herself right above her pubic bone. The uterus is smaller than most women imagine, about an inch and a half in length in a girl who has just reached puberty, about two and a half to three and a half inches in a woman who has menstruated but never had children, and four inches or so in a multiparous woman like Eleanor, a woman who has carried three children and suffered one miscarriage. In pregnant women, the pliant uterus expands, growing up out of the pelvis and finally, in the ninth month, reaching a woman's ribs. It crowds out the intestines and presses on the liver. It squeezes the bladder and shoves the stomach ever higher until it takes over the body, asserting its supremacy.

As a female embryo develops, her primordial uterus begins to stir in the fifth week, just when the heart begins to beat. Two thickenings called müllerian ducts arise within the developing embryo's body. In the sixth week, the two ducts approach each other, and a week later they join to form a single canal. The upper poles of these ducts become the oviducts, or tubes, and the fused segment becomes the uterus. By the third month, the passageway from the uterine fundus to the vagina is complete. By the sixth month, the vagina is patent, open and waiting. But for now it is the cervix, the neck of the uterus, that is our only concern.

Imagine the thick stump of Eleanor's cervix visible in the vaginal vault. Imagine a surgeon as she catches the end of the cervix with sutures to hold it steady, then takes a thin, sharp scalpel and carves out a cone like a dunce's cap. The peak of the cone is deep, almost reaching the internal os. The sides extend out, removing the entire end of the cervix. In the future when Eleanor returns for Pap tests, we will look into her vagina and see only this remnant, a carved-out V. The bulk of her large, often dilated cervix will be gone, but, we hope, so will the cancer.

Once removed, this cone-shaped wedge will be inspected by a

pathologist in minute detail. If there is no evidence that cancer cells have escaped—if there are no irregular cells seen under the microscope hiding in the small O of a vessel or lymph channel, waiting to be carried away through the body—Eleanor may be cured. If the cancer has spread beyond the borders of the cone, she will require a hysterectomy to eradicate any locus of errant cells: "hysterectomy," from the Greek *hystera,* meaning "womb," and *ek-tome,* meaning "excision."

When a woman's hormones surge and rage, she's often called hysterical, a disorder one old medical text from my collection defines as "a dysfunction of the nervous system characterized by numbness and tingling in the limbs and lips, convulsions, and perversion of morals and intellect." Because, according to this 1812 primer, doctors thought women suffered these symptoms more often than men, they blamed the uterus. Take out the uterus, medical science decided, and you could calm the woman. But the pejorative "hysterical" is inappropriate. The uterus is an innocent vessel; it produces no hormones. The ovaries, not the womb, are responsible for the chemical flux that might evoke the premenstrual or perimenopausal anxiety and moodiness that have often been labeled craziness or hysteria. Remove the uterus but leave the ovaries, and a woman will still produce a monthly egg, still experience estrogen and progesterone's monthly rise and fall. Without the uterus, there will be no menstrual blood and no receptacle in which a fertilized egg might grow, but a woman's days may still be rocked by her hormones' sometimes unpredictable shifts.

"Eleanor's cone biopsy went well," Emily said. "A great case."

After excising the cone-shaped piece of Eleanor's cervix, Emily controlled the bleeding and applied Gelfoam, a spongy material that helps seal any bleeding vessels, to the remaining nub. Finally she packed Eleanor's vagina with gauze. In twenty-four hours, Emily will remove the packing and inspect her surgical handiwork. "I wasn't worried about causing Eleanor any future childbearing problems—the incompetent cervix a large cone biopsy might cause—so I took a generous biopsy. The cervix that remained looked healthy," Emily said.

When she told me about the case, I listened with a fascination that had to do both with my regard for Eleanor and with my love for the twinned practices of surgery and medicine. Emily, like most doctors, wants to conquer disease, and she enjoys the well-oiled machinery of surgery, the right moves and correct guesses, the way the body and the tissues respond. The truth is, without respect for these exacting disciplines, no matter how much we care for our patients, not one of us would be able to do what we do. Loving the art of medicine as well as the body allows us to look beyond individual suffering to see the collective good. Knowing that there *is* a collective good, the discovery of new ways to cure, the possibility of restoring health gives us the strength we need to go forward and treat each patient as an individual. We can stand by the bedside of a suffering patient and tell her to hold on, to endure the treatments and the waiting. We can inflict necessary pain only if the patient agrees that the final outcome justifies the means.

After my day in the clinic ends, I take the elevator up to the eleventh floor to visit Eleanor.

She's sitting up in bed waiting for her husband, *The New York Times* spread over her blanket and a cup of gelatin on a tray in front of her. Small multicolored reading glasses perch halfway down her nose, and when she sees me her face becomes rosier, her mouth expands like a generous rubber band, her eyes scintillate.

"Hello!" she says and extends her left hand straight out to me. I've never felt more welcome.

Her right hand has intravenous tubing threaded under a clear plastic dressing and into a vein, and she rests this hand on the covers. She clears a space for me to sit down and pats the sheets beside her.

When I was in nursing school we learned never, never to sit on a patient's bed. Not only was this practice unclean—there might be germs on our uniforms, after all—it was also too familiar. When I graduated in 1972, nurses were supposed to carry out three main functions: observe patients, manage patients and act as their advocate within the hospital environment, and carry out orders and treatments skillfully and to the letter. We weren't supposed to get too close. We weren't supposed to reveal too much about ourselves or become overly involved with patients. Such lapses might affect our powers of impartial observation.

Once a nursing supervisor caught me sitting beside a terminally ill patient, holding his hand and listening instead of changing the sheets on the one empty bed in the room. She pulled me aside. "There's an unmade bed here," she said. "And you have two other patient rooms to finish." I didn't say it—I should have—but I thought it to myself: Aren't nurses supposed to tend patients, rather than their beds? After she huffed away, I used my own judgment, went back to my patient, and hoisted myself onto the bedclothes beside him. I just sat there. How else can you hold someone? How else can you accompany the dying or greet those newly awakened from the quick blank moment of anesthesia?

I sit on the bed in the space Eleanor has cleared by moving her legs. I tell her she looks fine, and she tries to make me believe that this operation was easier than she'd anticipated.

"Really, I hardly have any discomfort," she offers. "Well, some cramps once in a while. And I am a little tired."

For a while I stay with her as she makes faces at her Jell-O and occasionally takes a bite. I tell her I'm happy the cone biopsy is done with. That I hope this will be the end of her problems. Outside, the October afternoon dims quickly. In the parking lot, tall lights flare all at once, and the sky becomes a brilliant orange. As we watch, it blurs into gold. Then night comes like a huge pewter candle snuffer, and I close the drapes.

Usually I don't visit patients when they're in the hospital, other than a quick hello, an oh-what-a-beautiful-baby to an especially favorite patient on Labor and Delivery, or sometimes a brief head-in-the-door greeting to a patient the day after her surgery. Once a patient is hospitalized, she becomes the doctors' responsibility. Sometimes I wonder if I've become too much like a doctor—hasty, worried about fixing patients, overcome by the volume of paperwork, the reading and ongoing education it takes to keep pace with medical information—although I know many physicians who manage to find the time it takes to nurture patients.

When I was head nurse on the cancer ward, one of the oncologists and I made rounds every day. One morning, an old man dying of colon cancer stopped us before we could leave the room. He looked up at the doctor and asked, "Doc, am I dying?"

The oncologist walked to the bed and sat down next to the thin, blanketed ridge of the patient's legs. Holding both the patient's hands in his, the doctor said, "If you had a crystal ball, what would you see?"

"I'd see that I'm dying," the old man replied.

"You're right," the doctor said, still grasping the patient's skeletal hands. "Now, what can I do to help you get ready?"

How generous that doctor was. He didn't protect himself from the pain of speaking difficult truths. Sometimes a caring human presence *is* more potent than medicine. I decide to linger a few more minutes. A nurse arrives to check on Eleanor and adjust her IV.

"You know," Eleanor says, "suddenly I don't feel so good."

The nurse checks her blood pressure, glances at me with an *uh-oh* look, and leaves the room to call Emily. I stay with Eleanor.

When Emily arrives, I step out and she closes the curtain around Eleanor's bed. In a moment, Emily calls out.

"Wait here a second, OK?" she says. I hear a series of small sounds as Eleanor shifts her body, allows the resident to lift her sheets and check the pad between her legs. There's a few seconds of silence—Emily's murmur, something from Eleanor I can't hear. Emily comes quickly from behind the curtain and puts her hand on my arm in passing.

"Bleeding through the packing. Will you page the attending on call to my beeper?" She hurries from the room.

Eleanor's face is chalky with fear. I use her bedside phone to page the on-call gynecologist who's covering the clinic. "Please call Emily stat at beeper 0878," I say. I take Eleanor's reading glasses from her hand, roll the head of her bed down, and cover her with the thin blanket scrunched at her feet.

"What's happening?" she asks. For the first time, she looks frightened.

"It looks as though you're having some bleeding."

"Why would I be bleeding?"

"It's one of the complications of a cone biopsy," I reply. I don't tell her that the uterine arteries run beside the body of the uterus and alongside the cervix. If one of these branches is disturbed during the cone biopsy—a distinct possibility—the incidence of post-operative hemorrhage can be as high as 30 percent. If the bleeding is bad, women may require transfusion. This was one of the many risks listed on the permission form Eleanor signed, but maybe she didn't read it. Or perhaps she was afraid to ask questions, even when Emily went over the risks with her again.

"Oh, my God," Eleanor says and draws the blanket up under her chin.

Her whole body begins to quiver, and I stand beside her, soothing her arm and helping to tuck her blanket higher.

"It's going to be OK. You're in good hands. Emily will take care of you."

Eleanor looks small in the white sheets. Out of place.

"Am I going to die?" she asks me.

I hate this part of my job. Not the speaking of difficult truths but how, even when I don't know what a patient's outcome might be, I still have to act *sure* about things, relying only on an armful of facts, years of experience, and my gut feeling.

"No," I say, "you're *not* going to die."

Emily returns, her lab coat stark and fluorescent in the dimly lit room, as if she were an apparition moving closer, a good spirit.

"OK, Mrs. McCabe," she says, "we're taking you back to the OR."

The nurse calls Eleanor's husband while a nurse's aide arrives with a gurney. Emily and I help Eleanor slide over. I lift the IV tubing, loop it in place, and hang the plastic bag of fluid high on the stainless-steel pole. Emily asks, "Did you have anything to eat besides Jell-O, Eleanor?" as she pushes the stretcher, one hand on the frame and the other on her beeper. It goes off in a raucous series of high-pitched bleeps. She and the aide steer Eleanor out the door and down the hall.

"Good luck!" I call, but the disembodied sound of my words doesn't quite reach them.

Chapter 24

"I can't sleep, and my legs are fat," Lila says, sitting like a swollen gourd at the end of the table.

Lila looks ten years older than she did the last time I saw her. Her hair has grown out now—only the ends look russet under the clinic lights—and she wears no earrings. I remember her from her very first visit, before she knew she was pregnant, her vibrant red hair and outrageous hoops, her irreverent attitude, her almost boy-like body. Now, not even the baby tumbling around inside seems to give Lila any pleasure.

"Just take the damn baby out." She looks at me, and I see black smudges under her eyes where her mascara has run.

"Are you OK, Lila?" I ask, hoping she might actually answer me.

Lila ignores my question and looks around. She can't quite get used to being cared for, no matter how much we try. She still believes we forced her to come back to the clinic by sending Rita after her.

It took Rita a few weeks to track down Lila and Charles, but she finally found them staying with another couple, one of Charles's friends and his girlfriend. Lila was the youngest and the least able to defend herself, in spite of her years of street education, so the three of them decided that Lila should become their maid. She cleaned and cooked for them, and they made her hand over her welfare check as rent.

When Rita knocked on the apartment door on a tip from another girl, Lila appeared carrying a broom. Although she looked angry and barely spoke, she did let Rita in.

"I don't need to come to the clinic so much," Lila said.

"Yes, you do," Rita answered, and told her to come in the next day at nine in the morning.

"I can't," Lila protested. She told Rita she had to make breakfast, clean the dishes, vacuum, and dust every morning before ten. Then, while Charles and his friend went out, Lila and the other girl sat and watched TV until lunchtime, when Lila had to make sandwiches. Yes, Charles was shoving her around, she confessed, and Rita probed until she learned that he was also tempting Lila with cocaine, her drug-of-choice payment for being the live-in housekeeper. Charles and his friends didn't let her go to the clinic; in fact, they rarely left her alone. The morning Rita arrived was one of the exceptions. Charles and his friends had gone out to buy doughnuts.

"I mean it," Lila snarls at me. "Take it out."

By thirty-four or thirty-five weeks of pregnancy most women want to deliver and get back to normal, even though the baby's not quite ready—not until thirty-seven weeks are the lungs and kidneys mature enough to withstand life outside the uterus without risk. Lila's no different. She wants to deliver and be done with it, too. She's fed up right on schedule.

When Lila finally reappeared at the clinic, her belly was measuring smaller than it should have. One of the residents did an ultrasound and found that the baby's growth was on schedule but the placenta was grade two, pocked here and there with calcium deposits, an aging condition caused by Lila's cigarettes. The baby's ribs showed up like small white wishbones, and, Lila said, its legs looked like skinny sticks poking straight out. The resident saw that Lila's baby was a girl. When Lila heard this, she beamed. "Won't Charles be happy," she said.

Last week the drug counselor met with Lila and asked for a

urine screen. Again she explained that the baby would be taken away if Lila or her newborn tested positive for drugs at the time of delivery. Lila, the social worker told us, said she was clean.

Soon we'll begin monitoring Lila's unborn baby girl every week. If the baby's heart rate increases appropriately when the baby moves, we'll know enough oxygen is filtering through the aging placenta. Lila finds all this attention annoying rather than reassuring. She hasn't settled on a name yet, but Charles, overjoyed that he would now have both a boy and a girl, suggested the name Angel. Lila said that made her think of dead babies. Anyway, she protested on the days she was angry with Charles, this is *my* baby.

Today, it seems as if Lila and I have come to an impasse in our relationship. My patience is worn thin, and it's almost impossible for me to deal with her. In spite of myself, I'm beginning to wonder if Lila doesn't bring some of this hardship on herself. After months of trying to cajole and encourage her, I've had it with her little-girl attitude and her apparent lack of involvement with this pregnancy. She's been abandoned by her parents, ignored by the system, and victimized by her boyfriend. I try to remember that she doesn't need me to turn against her, too.

At the moment, I don't think she likes me either. She says she likes Yanna better. Yanna, like Lila, has a way of avoiding issues.

"Yanna told me I didn't *have* to do my fetal movement counts every day," Lila whines.

"Counting your baby's movements is extremely important. If the baby's not moving well, it could mean there's a problem. Your placenta has been affected by smoking and drugs."

"I fall asleep when I count."

"Then count for half an hour."

"I have to cook for Charles and them before six."

"Tell Charles to cook for himself."

"Right, you want me to get beat?"

"How about if I call Meg and we get you into the battered women's shelter?"

"How will Charles know when to come to the hospital? I mean, he's *gotta* be there."

"If Charles hits you, will he hit the baby?"

Lila looks away and pumps her leg up and down. "I can't stand this backache," she says. "Take the baby out."

"It's too early. If the baby's born now, she could have trouble breathing. She might need a respirator."

"She *won't.* Anyhow, I don't care what happens. I just want it over." Her voice ricochets against the white enamel cabinets and bounces off the posters listing the various types of birth control: the pill, IUDs, diaphragms, Depo-Provera injections, Norplant, condoms, foam.

Part of me is disgusted with Lila. She looks unkempt, her teeth look as though they haven't been brushed in a few days, and she's making stupid faces, curling up her lip or sticking out her tongue when she thinks I can't see. She seems to have total disregard for her baby. I feel myself becoming insensitive, merciless.

"Lie down, Lila," I growl. "I have to check your cervix."

I don't look at her, and she looks at the wall. She's also angry that I made Charles stay in the waiting room. First I was shocked that he actually came with Lila for a visit. Then I told him I wanted Lila to come into the exam room by herself. Charles had sunglasses on so I couldn't see his eyes, but I know he looked me up and down. In the brief glimpse I had of him, he looked older than twenty-eight. Tough. His jaw was square and clean-shaven, pitted with old acne scars. His body was square, too, and I could see he was slightly bowlegged with too-long pants bunched above his high-top sneakers. Then he turned away, smacking a pack of cigarettes, *tok tok tok,* into his open palm.

Lila's cervix is rich with hormones. My fingertip reaches the internal os, the cervical opening. Lila is a fingertip dilated, a somewhat unusual finding in a primip, a woman having her first baby. She's not having any contractions, she tells me. Nevertheless, her cervix is changing, ripening. It's something to watch.

"Are you doing any coke?"

Lila looks furious. "None of your goddamn business," she spits.

"It is my business if you put yourself into labor. If you have a premature baby who dies."

"I'm thirty-five weeks," Lila says, sitting up. "Thirty-*five* weeks. That's enough. My mother had me when I was thirty-*four* weeks! See?"

My hands are wrinkled from wearing latex gloves all day, putting them on, double-gloving, peeling them off, washing my hands. I'm hot. The colder it gets outside, the more heat blasts through the clinic and no one seems to be able to regulate it. I'm tired of dealing with patients who don't speak English but laugh at my attempts to speak their language. I'm sick of patients who are poor, who are undereducated, who hit their children, who do drugs. I'm tired of women who have five or six abortions as a way of birth control, tired of women who go ahead and have babies they don't want and then neglect them, tired of men who hit their girlfriends. I'm tired of men who take great pride in getting their girlfriends pregnant but take no responsibility for their offspring. I'm tired of hearing about no money for rent, no money for food.

Lila's tired, too. She's tired of women like me who waltz in the door and tell her to eat right, do right, and pay attention to this lump in her belly when she can't find a safe place to live and can't get anyone to validate her existence. She's tired of trying to call her father only to have the phone hung up in her ear, tired of wondering where her mother is and why she left. She's tired of waiting on a man, thinking it will get him to love her when all it does is make him despise her. She's tired of wearing the same pair of black stretch pants every day, tired of waking up to no heat, no plans, a future as dry and dismal as this November's falling leaves.

Today it's easier for Lila to hate me than to change her life. Today it's easier for me to blame Lila than it is to work with her. It's easier to think *Let her have a premature baby.* It's tempting to believe that patients like Lila deserve everything they get: the men who mistreat them, the bus drivers who close doors in their faces, the caregivers who don't listen to them.

I lean against the wall and look at Lila. I arrange my face so it doesn't reveal what I'm thinking, and just changing my expression, I notice, makes me feel a bit better. Lila has taken a time out too. She folds her hands and takes a deep breath, and her face loses that hard edge. We're both having second thoughts, regrouping. We're both so burned out we can hardly talk without crying.

"You don't understand," she says to me. "I'm *really* trying."

"I know," I say. "I'd like to help in any way I can." We both know it's mostly up to her.

She's quiet for a moment, then asks when she has to come back.

"Next week. In the meantime, call if you have any problems or any contractions or if the baby's not moving well, OK? Even in the middle of the night." I bend over backward to make sure Lila knows we're available.

"OK." Lila glances at me briefly and heaves herself off the table, holding her sides. I steady her with a hand on her shoulder. When I give her the slip of paper for a return appointment, our hands touch briefly. Her skin feels soft and warm.

In spite of myself, I know I'll think about Lila every day. When I go grocery shopping and load boxes of cereal and big cans of soup into my basket, I'll wonder if she has enough to eat. When one of my children says something unexpected and endearing and my heart soars with love for them, I'll wonder who loves Lila.

When I was her age, I hadn't discovered boys. Instead, I loved horses. While other fifteen-year-old girls played spin the bottle in their parents' basements, I drew pictures of wild stallions running and plunging over meadows filled with flowers and vines. I drew colts with spindly legs too long for their bodies. I imagined I had my own horse, a black stallion named Faker, and sometimes when the school bus whizzed down the highway, I'd look out the window and see myself riding him as he galloped along with his big, ground-eating strides. I could go anywhere. I never had any doubt.

When I became a young mother, I learned how difficult it was to fulfill those dreams. As my own children grew, I watched them develop inside the life I had made for them, one in which they were loved and yet their spirits were damped by divorce, poverty, and the ghost of a mother who drove them from baby-sitter to baby-sitter so she could work and go to school and then study until three in the morning, who wanted to graduate from nursing school and support them, who wondered how she could ever enable them to fulfill dreams of their own.

I want to ask Lila what *she* imagines, what she longs for. I wish I could hug her and rock her, let her cry against me for as long as it takes. When I see Lila, I see all the children who must make their own way. I see the women who have fashioned insufficient worlds for them and yet done the best they can. I want to rescue Lila, with one wave of my hand, from Charles and his friends, from the cramped existence that Lila, so desperate to belong, accepts.

But it's impossible for any of us to rescue our patients. While there are plenty of boundaries to break, there are also boundaries to keep and lines over which we cannot step. If we can't locate the place where we end and our patients begin, our clinical instincts can become clouded and inaccurate, our wishes can preempt theirs. Yet taken too far, this division is deadening. Then it becomes too painful to empathize with patients, too easy to sweep them into a corner, labeled and depersonalized. Somewhere, I know, there is a balance point.

Before Lila goes I stop her for a moment, holding her shoulders firmly. For a second she leans into my grasp, and we look at each other. She almost begins to cry, and I almost hold her, like the mother she doesn't have, and comfort her.

Chapter 25

"I'm taking a walk," I announced at lunchtime one day about four years ago. Nina was an intern then, still unsure of her skills and not settled into the clinic routine. One of the older residents looked at her and said, "Cortney walks in the cemetery." The resident drew out the word "ce-me-ter-y" and waggled his fingers in Nina's face.

"Great," she replied. "Can I go too?"

Of all the residents who have come and gone from the clinic, Nina's my favorite. Almond-eyed and perpetually relaxed, she's half Korean, bluntly honest, and funny. When she's exhausted from being on call, she sleeps unashamedly in her chair, her body limp and her mouth open, clean as a cat's. When she's awake, she's interested in the world and absolutely unflappable in an emergency. We became friends on our first walk, and since then we've walked in the huge cemetery across the street from the big brick hospital whenever we can, usually just a quick fifteen minutes at lunch or, once in a while, a stroll after work. We like to walk in the cemetery in spring, when the new grass pushes up around the headstones, and in early winter, like now, when the trees have shed their leaves and starlings fly up from the hedges. The white snow and stark gray stones are primeval; then, the sun strikes them like a match.

We like to read the names on the stones and make up stories

about the lives of those who lie beneath. When we walk, we don't talk about work. Instead we talk about our childhoods and our parents or about books we're reading, women's issues, and politics. A walk in the cemetery certainly puts things into perspective.

We know where the huge oak trees hide us from view, where the weeping cherries will turn hazy green next spring, casting their shadows over the pond that is home to Canada geese raising their goslings and turtles sunning themselves on large flat rocks, plopping into the water one by one as we go by.

We've seen white herons and groundhogs, flying squirrels and raccoons and thin coppery fish that dart through the pond weeds. Crows have taken up residence here as well, and when they perch on top of gravestones against the cobalt sky their combined silhouettes are ominous.

"It's a perfect cemetery," Nina says, shuffling along, her black hair blown by the chilly wind.

We like to go up the front steps of the few mausoleums to peer through their foggy front windows at the paintings on the glass inside. When the sun is just right, the pictures light up: carnelian and yellow flowers blooming at the base of a cross. Beyond these, there are a Jewish section, an Arab section, a Japanese section, and a Greek section. There's even a pauper's field, where a series of unmarked depressions lies in perfect symmetry, some of the sunken graves big as a man, some tiny as a child.

We prefer gravestones that have information on them, usually the older ones. We like knowing that Evva had been the wife of Harold, that her soul was called to God on the third day of May in 1889, when she was thirty-nine years, two months, and twelve days old. When we looked for Harold's plot, we found that he'd married again. Mary, Harold's second wife, lay nearby, and May, his third and last wife, outlived him by ten years and ten days.

One spring we stumbled across the oldest section in the cemetery, where a line of reverends was buried in the late 1700s. Their stones were thin, but the old writing was crisp and distinct. *Let's talk of graves, and worms and epitaphs.* Hovering over one stone was a death's-head, the winged, blank-eyed face that looked more like a skull. Just the right stone for a rubbing.

Nina and I hauled tape and blocks of black rubbing wax, sheets of tough paper, and newspapers that we could sit on, to the end of Reverends' Row. Our white coats fluttering in the breeze, we rubbed and rubbed, watching the Old English letters with their curly tails reappear beneath our hands. "After all this time," Nina said.

Most of all, we like to find the mementos left by the living on the graves of their loved ones: letters and cards wrapped in plastic bags to protect them from the weather, dishes of food and toy metal cars, Halloween masks and bags of candy corn that melt in the rain or are eaten by ghosts, flowers wrapped in silver foil that say "Wonderful Mom" or "Dear Sister," an infant's cup, a circle of pennies, tinsel that sparkles on nearby trees until it curls up in the intense summer sun. We always look for gifts on the graves of our patients.

Kelly is buried in the far end of the cemetery on a bit of an incline overlooking the dirt road before the duck pond. Her headstone is still black and shiny with a carving of a rose over her name. Underneath, it says, "Kelly, our beloved daughter, who loved life." Kelly was seventeen. She and her boyfriend and two others died in a house fire. When I see Kelly's grave, I'm reminded, sharply, that every one of our patients has a family. I wonder why it must sometimes be death that unites them.

Kelly's family has remembered every holiday, no matter how small. Every few months her grave decorations change, reflecting the seasons and the cyclical celebrations to which we humans cling. Nina and I have walked in the cemetery for four years. Little by little, the gifts and the keepsakes left on Kelly's grave are dwindling.

Today we've come to the cemetery at lunchtime. We barely have ten minutes left before we have to go back and face the whirlwind clinic afternoon. I'm going to miss Nina, who will graduate next June and begin a new life. I'm old enough to be her mother. Nevertheless, we talk about things I've never discussed with my children: what it will be like to be old; how strange it will be to leave this earth and our loved ones behind; what we want the purpose of our lives to be.

Sometimes she teases me. "Come work with me in Colorado," she says. "Leave the clinic behind." We turn to trudge up the hill toward the road. As we walk, she pulls a paper out of her coat pocket and opens it.

"I got Eleanor's cone biopsy results. Emily hasn't seen them yet." Nina and Emily have changed services. For the next few months Emily will be up in Labor and Delivery, and Nina will be in the clinic.

We stop walking, and she gives me the paper. I shield my eyes from the sun and the white glare that bounces off the page, making the small black letters even harder to read. I recognize that tightening in my stomach that accompanies the revelation of any unknown, but there's something about the way the pathology report opens like a letter that's even more exciting, as if I were reading someone else's mail. In a way I am. Nina knows, I will know, and soon Eleanor will know just what her body has revealed.

Microinvasive cervical cancer. The three words make one short stab across the page, which I refold in thirds and hand back to Nina. Poor Eleanor. First she bled and had to be taken back to the OR to be resutured, and now we learn that the abnormal cells on her cervix have continued their silent, sneaky proliferation in spite of our interventions. This means that Eleanor must have a hysterectomy. But that loss will save her life, according to the statistics, those cold numbers upon which we must finally base our decisions and our recommendations.

The cone biopsy specimen was sliced into more than fifty sections—the more samples the pathologist sees, the more likely he will be able to make a correct diagnosis. He would have studied the different sections one by one, each slide an infinitesimal cut deeper into the cervical tissue. It's a beautiful cold day. We walk back in silence.

When we enter the clinic, squinting in the artificial atmosphere and warmed by heat pouring from the ceiling vents, Nina and I each pick up a chart and get to work. I go into room 2 with a certain lightness, a willingness to listen and respond. There's something about our walks that centers me. I find I have more tolerance for our patients, more stamina to deal with the hundred interruptions and the yards of red tape. When I've seen the granite death's-head that looks like a grinning skull, I'm grateful to feel the outline of a baby's body through a stretched-thin abdomen. When I see the lovely faces of young girls melt into the seasoned faces of women and see my own face changing every day in the mirror, I know things are as they should be. I feel my soul honed by life.

Without the promise of death, I would find no poignancy in beauty or desire. Without my walk in the cemetery, the wonderful fresh faces of newborns would become commonplace, and the naïveté of our clinic teenagers would cloy, turning my day into a drudgery of service.

Emily will call Eleanor, and Eleanor will have her uterus removed, the end of one phase of her life and the beginning of another. Change is all there is in the clinic, a universe held not by Atlas on his back but by Venus on hers. Sometimes change comes with rejoicing, other times with suffering—but it always comes. Otherwise there'd be no point in memory, even less in hope.

Chapter 26

The words a woman uses to define herself are important. Some-times they reveal who she is. Other times, they serve to conceal her identity. In the clinic, I might ask a woman, "So, tell me about your-self." She might say, "I'm always in pain" or "I'm married with two children." If I ask a patient to tell me what's going on, she might reply, "Nothing," or she might growl, "I'm tired and cranky." But I want to know more about my patients. What metaphor might a woman invent for her life? What myth does she create when she tells others her story? How does she re-create the universal within the borders of her own experience, within the confines of her own body? I had asked Joanna to make a list of words that described who she is, not adjectives such as "tired" but verbs and nouns. Ac-tion words; concrete words to summon up the truth about Joanna and perhaps to unveil, at last, the emptiness in her soul.

I first came across this exercise when I attended a medical hu-manities conference in a small Ohio town not too far away from where Joanna's father lives. Two actors conducted a series of work-shops designed to pare away our pretenses and reveal our char-acters, enabling us to relate more personally with our patients. One night they handed out sheets of paper, numbered 1 to 25 for the twenty-five people in our group. Then they asked us each to write a list of nouns and verbs that described who we were. Write quickly, they said, fifty words at least. Our lists were collected and redistributed anonymously. Take the list you've received, they said, and make up a few sentences about that person, intuiting what that person is like from the words he or she has chosen. Then we read our descriptions aloud.

My list landed in the hands of a young woman with clouds of long red hair. "I have number four," she said. Then she read her impression of the woman behind all the words I had written, words such as *run, animal, dream, death, birth, wander, savor, wonder, magic, tears.*

"Many words, nouns, not roles," she read. "Unexpected, puzzling, written quickly. Contradictions, demands. Reminds me of a spelling list, a grocery list, reminds me that we're all very complex. Reminds me of a stained-glass window or a mosaic. This is a woman who juggles many worlds but is connected in sisterhood to nature, to *place* in the world. Mystery of the sacred ordinary, of womanhood, of the sexes, of many directions, of the story."

Her interpretation stunned me. I felt as if she knew not the superficial me sitting somewhat anxiously across the room from her but the particular me that had evolved from my childhood, my adolescence, my triumphs and mistakes, to become *me,* the person I understand myself to be. *That's what I want to know about my patients,* I thought then. That's what I want them to understand about themselves.

Tonight Joanna wears black trousers and a red jacket. Black boots with high, thin heels. Splashes of color on her face. Red lips, red cheeks. And red fingernails that look like rose petals at the ends of her slender fingers. *Sunrise,* I think to myself. *Gazelle.*

"Come on in," I say. "Let's go into room three."

Joanna is, once more, the last patient of the evening. My assistant locks up the cabinets and puts away the basket of blood-drawing equipment. "Will you need anything else?" she asks me. When she leaves, Joanna and I are the only ones there. Nevertheless, I close the door behind us. Soon enough the housekeeper will be coming through, pushing his cart with its spidery gray mops and metal garbage drums.

"I did what you suggested," Joanna says as soon as she sits down. In spite of the color on her cheeks, her face looks drawn. "Whenever David wanted to make love and I didn't, I tried to say something."

"How did it go?" I ask, pulling my rolling stool up in front of Joanna's chair.

"I couldn't get the words out." Her red lips smile at me, but she furrows her brow like a puzzled child. "A couple of times, when I tried to say, 'Not now,' I couldn't talk." She looks away. "Actually, I usually just started to cry."

I wait a full minute. I think she may begin to cry now as well, but she doesn't. Inside my head I count, *One and two and three,* all the way to sixty.

"What did David do?"

She takes a breath and says, "He was wonderful. He kept asking me what was wrong. He kept telling me that he loved me. That everything would be OK."

"Were you able to tell him what was wrong?"

"If I *knew,* I would have told him. I didn't think I could just say, 'Well, I don't want to have sex anymore, that's all.'"

"What do you think would happen if you did say that?"

Joanna looks down at her toes. She taps them up and down on the hard linoleum floor. "He'd think I didn't love him."

"Are you worried that if you don't have sex with him, he'll stop loving you?"

"I feel like . . . well, maybe I feel like sex is part of the deal."

I hesitate a minute. "Do you and David talk about other things that concern you?"

"When I was crying, he seemed hurt to think that there was anything I *couldn't* talk to him about, you know? He talked about how it was in Italy—remember, I told you? He said I seemed happier then. That I talked about a lot of things then." She hugs her knees, leans forward.

"Joanna," I say. "I wonder if David realizes how sad you are?" What I mean is *Joanna, do you realize how sad you are?*

The light on Joanna's skin changes from a translucent blush to an opaque mask, the way candle wax does when it drips slowly onto the tablecloth and, while you watch, becomes fixed and cloudy.

"Am I?" she asks. "I don't know."

She pushes back her hair. Her earrings are small black onyx buttons. In the next exam room, I hear the creak of the housekeeper's cart, then the damp smack of his mop.

I'm sure Joanna never told David that she'd slept with that other man. I wonder if that omission places an additional barrier between them. Some people feel that confessing infidelities simply causes unnecessary pain. Others have to get everything out in the open or they can't go forward emotionally.

"What is it, do you think, that makes it difficult for you to talk to David about sex?"

Joanna doesn't seem to hear me. She takes her word list, folded and folded again, out of her pocket. Changing the subject, I think to myself. Or maybe she's finally getting around to it.

"Look at my words," she says.

I unfold the paper and read Joanna's looping, fine handwriting. *Secret,* the column begins. Then *sun, canvas. Swim, painter,* and *villa.* The wonderful life in Italy, far away from Joanna's childhood in Ohio. The hours of painting, the sun coming through the window of the villa where Joanna and David fell in love. *Brush, lemon, raspberry.* Then, the emergence of some terrible event, Joanna's inability to shout out her unhappiness. I read *soul, crawl, fingers, child, mother, car, forget.*

I explain the exercise, how I'd like to make a copy of her list so I can write a brief impression of the woman these nouns and verbs might represent. I want Joanna to trust me, so I tell her about the words I chose and I paraphrase what the young red-haired woman wrote about me—more than I've ever revealed, perhaps, to any patient. Sometimes it's not necessary for patients to know much about me. Other times, it is. If I don't expose something of myself to Joanna at this point, our discussion might end. Patients probably know more about me than I realize anyway. Some of them have been coming to the clinic for all the years I've worked here.

Haven't they seen me age, seen me on days when I'm tired and short-tempered or on days when I'm willing to roll back and talk, laugh with them about our common experiences?

"I liked doing the list," Joanna says. "I even thought about asking David to make one." We both smile.

As we sit, waiting to see where this conversation will take us, Joanna rubs her hands together, almost wringing them. I hear the muted, repetitive *swoosh* of the housekeeper's mop as he begins cleaning, and, louder, the rasp of Joanna's palms, the click of her rings. The clinic is so still that all sounds echo.

"So," she says. "It's normal for a woman not to have an orgasm so easily or not to want to have sex?"

Joanna wants to stay focused on the clinical and avoid the emotional. She still longs to believe that it's her body that's somehow broken or abnormal and needs to be fixed.

"It depends," I say, and I repeat the information I gave her once before. Because I know that patients aren't always ready to hear things the first time around, I don't mind this repetition. It gives me a chance to reframe the words, approach the subject in a different way.

"Most women fall into the middle range. They feel the desire for sex at least occasionally, and most require direct stimulation of the clitoris, sometimes for a prolonged period of time, in order to reach orgasm. In some women's experience, orgasm is difficult to achieve under any circumstances. On the other end of the spectrum are women who require little stimulation and can experience multiple orgasms."

There are different stages of sexual response, and although Joanna can reach a climax, it seems that for her all the stages are blunted. Tonight, she says she no longer feels *desire,* that tingly feeling that's difficult to describe but serves to stimulate the changes in a woman's body that prepare it for sex. The vagina lubricates and actually expands. The nipples become more sensitive, and the breasts feel as if they're swelling. Then, with continued stimulation, a woman's level of excitement rises, crescendos to a peak. As she nears orgasm, her muscles tense, her heartbeat increases. The release of that tension, the climax, is the final stage in sexual responsiveness, like climbing up the mountain and allowing yourself to fall off. But there are wide variations in the way women experience those steps. Joanna's body is capable of orgasm. It's her spirit that can't let go.

"Well," Joanna says, "for me, it's like I'm not there. Like my body doesn't *feel* anything."

In the next room, the housekeeper scrapes the metal wastebasket across the floor. Then he turns the water on and off.

"Maybe I'm depressed," she says. "Maybe I should have called that therapist."

Yes, I think. *Here it is.*

Joanna looks at me, and as she talks she raises her hands in the air as if she's pleading with me or making a point. "I mean, I get dressed and go to work and eat and everything. It's not like I'm *so* depressed I can't function. But sometimes isn't depression on the inside?" She touches her heart, and her eyes get shiny. I'm feeling such sadness for Joanna that my eyes tear as well.

I reach over and place the palm of my hand on her arm. "Joanna, do you ever feel so depressed that you think about hurting yourself?" This question may seem to come out of nowhere, but I've learned that even the slightest admission of depression requires investigation. Patients contemplating suicide often answer this inquiry honestly. "Yes," women have said to me, "I even know how I would do it."

"No," she says, wiping her eyes. "No, I would *never* do that. It's just that I feel this way *all the time.*"

Joanna lowers her head, and I see her shoulders rise and fall. I see the tears that drop down to her hands as they rest quietly on her knees, as if part of her body is finally able to grieve. The rest is separated away, locked in some room that Joanna keeps hidden under the huge gray blanket of silence that she must drag around from place to place: *secret, fingers, child, forget.* Her message couldn't be more clear.

"Joanna," I say, and move my rolling stool closer to her chair. I know I'm negotiating treacherous ground. I tighten my grasp on her arm.

"I'm going to ask you the same question I've asked before. If you don't want to answer, that's OK, but I want to ask you again. So many women have been sexually abused, in childhood or as adults. I always ask my patients if they're one of those women."

Sometimes these women only nod their heads yes in response to my question and say no more. Other women seem relieved, as if someone has finally permitted them to speak. Many women don't wait for my question at all but offer their anguish spontaneously and rapidly, as if the words have been dammed up too long and must erupt as soon as the exam room door is closed. Then there are women like Joanna. For them, abuse is a figure in a dream or a touch that can't quite be recalled. Sometimes one image returns, and when that image is pulled from the dank cellar of the past, all the others follow, rushing up the stairs.

Joanna begins to sob noiselessly, her lips held tightly closed, her body rocking with every breath, a pantomime of grief. The memory that causes Joanna such pain is stuck deep in the recesses of her body. I wonder if this memory resides in her vagina or dwells in her hands. I wonder if it circles her breasts or pries open the corners of her mouth.

I wonder who it was. I wonder when it happened. The facts are staggering. There are millions who have endured childhood abuse, both males and females, but girls are victimized three times as often as boys. If a women was raped in childhood, her attacker was most likely a family member or friend. And rape isn't the only crime. As many as one woman out of four has been sexually accosted in *some* way before the age of fourteen. There are forcing and touching, kissing and tickling, sodomy and humiliation. There's a wide range of emotional injuries that might not include the physical yet can be just as damaging. Whatever it is, abuse always starts with one little act. A look. A stealthy touch. A secret. A mood in the room that changes when a certain person walks in.

"It's so silly," Joanna says, trying to speak, trying to sit up straight. "It wasn't a big deal. I don't even know why I'm crying."

"It doesn't matter what it was," I say. "What matters is that it wasn't your fault. What matters is how it has affected your life."

Joanna looks up at the ceiling, opening her eyes wide to dry them, breathing through her mouth to slow her heart. Every once in a while her control weakens and she sobs or she closes her eyes tight and grimaces. Her shoulders are steel, her hands are cold flint, and her arm is granite under my palm. That's how much energy it takes for her body to repress its hundred denied emotions.

"Do you want to tell me about it?" I ask.

Chapter 27

There is something about two women face-to-face in a small room that allows confession, or perhaps there is something in the nature of sorrow that longs to be shared. When a woman speaks, I catch hold of her words as if they were silken threads. Slowly I gather them in, braiding the strands and hoping to create something tangible just by listening.

When Joanna is able, she begins.

"My mother's brother . . . my Uncle Dan. He lived down the street from us from the time I was four until I was maybe thirteen. His two daughters were my favorite cousins. He was my favorite uncle."

Joanna looks up at me and smiles. "He taught me how to swim underwater, you know, how to hold my breath and keep my eyes open. He told me once that sleeping with a pillow was bad for your posture, so for two weeks I tried to sleep without one, flat on the mattress. Anything to be like him. In the summer, he'd take all of us kids out for ice cream. He had a car with a big backseat, and we'd all scrunch down on the floor and talk while Uncle Dan drove. He used to come over to my house all the time. To watch TV, to hang out with my mom. Or I'd be down at their house, waiting for his kids to finish dinner so we could play. But after a while, it was really Uncle Dan that I wanted to see."

I picture Joanna and her uncle at the beach. Her slim body underwater, streaking like a minnow in his powerful wake. She must have believed that his trespass was her fault, that her admiration brought it on.

"When did it start?" I ask.

Joanna hunches her shoulders and squeezes her eyes shut. "I don't *remember.* I don't remember much of anything except a few flashes, like movie scenes or bits of something he said. I know he would baby-sit for me and my brother once in a while. He would let me sit in the front seat sometimes when all of us went for a ride."

"I have a friend who was abused by a family member too," I say. "She remembers sounds and textures more than actual events."

"I remember that he used to bring big bags of pretzels for me. I remember the salty taste and how the bag crackled when I reached in. He used to hold it on his lap and then he'd say, 'Come on, don't you want another pretzel?' He used to call me his baby."

"What else did he do?"

Joanna sits up straight, covers her face. I haven't taken my hand from her arm, and now I feel her trembling. My heart is pounding.

"Oh, my God, when I think of what *I* did. I used to flirt with him. If he didn't pay attention to me, I'd pout and slam my bedroom door." She looks at me. "He never *hurt* me. I always thought he loved me."

"My friend said that too—that for a long time she felt guilty. She told me that part of her was horrified by what this family friend had done, but another part of her had enjoyed it. Now she knows that was a normal response."

"He'd rub me. I'd lie on my bed in my nightie, and he'd rub me down there and rub and rub. I always thought that must be why it takes me so long to have an orgasm. I always thought my uncle *trained* me that way." She pounds her fist on her thigh. Under my hand, her arm tightens and releases, tightens and releases. She raises her hand and touches two fingers to her forehead, as if she might massage the memories away.

"When I was really little, I'd jump up and down on my bed and he'd tell me to take my panties off, then he'd sit on the floor and watch me. I couldn't see what he was doing, but I knew he was doing something to himself. His face would get ugly. Once my brother came in, and Uncle Dan screamed at him to get out and leave me alone. I remember being upset because my brother wasn't bothering me at all. I couldn't stop jumping until my uncle told me. 'Stop now, you'll get dizzy and fall,' he'd say, like I was doing something wrong. Then he'd say, 'Don't tell anyone, OK, baby?' Every time I'd see him, he'd get me alone and say, 'You didn't tell anyone about our game, did you?'

"One time when my parents' car was broken, he drove my mother and father somewhere, to the doctor or something. They went in, and I waited in the car with him. He had a newspaper, and he put it over his lap, then he took my hand and put it under the paper. I just sat there and watched his face get uglier and uglier. Then I saw my dad walking toward the car, and I thought he'd come back to save me, that he *knew.* When Uncle Dan saw him, he grabbed some tissues and shoved them under the paper. My hand was sticky all over. I remember the smell, dusty and nauseating. I remember the car seats, too. They were dark green. Like fake velvet."

"Did your father notice what was going on?" I ask.

"No, I don't think so. He came back to tell us my mom's visit would take longer than they thought. He didn't want to inconvenience Dan or make me worry."

"Then your dad walked away?"

"Yup. He walked away, and my uncle folded up the paper and pushed me over to the other side of the car. 'This is our secret,' he said. 'Right?' "

———

When I was twelve, my parents and I moved from Pennsylvania to our white Colonial house in Connecticut. The first summer we were there, some of my parents' old neighborhood friends came up to visit. One couple stayed for a week. The woman was short and plump, her hair rolled tight in a bun at the nape of her neck, and when she chewed gum, she snapped it, a habit my mother hated. Her husband was blond, smooth-faced, and young-looking. He wore slim, freshly ironed shirts tucked into chinos, and his belt buckle was always placed precisely in the middle of his waist, like a military man's, his buckle in line with his shirt buttons and fly. They had one son, whom they disciplined severely. If he didn't finish his dinner, he'd sit for what seemed like hours waiting to be excused, the food cold and lumpy on the plate before him.

The first few days of their visit, the man ignored me. On the third day, he and I were sitting on the patio surrounded by summer—my mother's bleeding hearts drooping in the garden and the sweet scent of the cut grass left behind by my dad's lawn mower. We were talking about my new braces, the shiny wires I hated so much that I refused to smile. "No, no," our visitor said to me. "You're too pretty to keep your lips pinched together. You should lick your lips, then let them come apart a little, like this." He showed me, and I copied him. Lick my lips, upper first, then lower. Close the lips, then relax them so they parted, letting only the tips of my front teeth show through. Like a movie star. "That's it," he said. I was embarrassed. I didn't want him to notice how my front teeth stuck out or how, when my mouth was closed, I still looked bucktoothed. Maybe, I reasoned, he was trying to help me. When I practiced before the mirror, lips moistly parted as he suggested, I didn't look so much like a rabbit.

The day before they left, the man and I were once again in the backyard. His wife was packing, chatting with my mother in the upstairs guest room. Their voices floated from the open window and diffused into the hot August air. My dad was watering the grass out front. A zillion cicadas were humming. I could hear the water from the hose as it occasionally hit the whitewashed siding, slapping and clattering before my dad would redirect the spray. I was wearing white shorts and a white cotton top. I had just taken a bath, and I smelled clean. I felt clean. Squeaky. Fresh.

This man and I stood together. I didn't know what to talk about. Breaking the silence, he complimented me on the way I'd learned to pout. I didn't understand what he meant. Then he kissed me, his mouth thick against mine. He pushed his tongue through my lips, urged it forward until I felt its bulk, warm and insistent. I pulled away, startled and ashamed. I remembered how, when my friends and I were nine or ten, we'd dared each other to touch tongues. We'd draw closer, our tongues stuck out until the tips touched and we felt that awful, animal softness, a contact both electric and repulsive. Then we would squeal and separate, shake our heads and pretend to spit.

The visitor man laughed and walked away. I felt dirty and suddenly wiser. Grown up.

Sometime later, my parents and I were driving in the car. I leaned over the seat and said, "You know when the Millers were here the other day?" Yes, they said. What about it? "Well," I said, "when Mr. Miller kissed me good-bye he put his tongue in my mouth. Isn't that weird?" My father kept driving. My mother folded her gloves on top of her pocketbook and unfolded them again. They didn't say anything. Why, I wondered, didn't they say *something*? Why didn't they condemn his act, say he was *wrong*, reassure me that what had happened was his fault, not mine? But they did do something. We never saw the Millers again. A family that had once been numbered among my parents' good friends was simply stricken from the list. No phone calls. No Christmas or birthday cards. I never heard their names again.

That was my earliest encounter with abuse, the first time I learned how easy it is to become the prey and how difficult it is to bring that experience into focus. The unexpected kiss was a mere ripple, something that served to make me vigilant. But it was nothing, *nothing* like what happened to Joanna.

————————

She sits up straight, her hands still resting on her lap. Her eyes are clear, her lids red-rimmed and puffy. She looks not quite composed but emotionally removed, as if she has cut herself in two and what she says has no connection to her body. Only occasionally does her memory become visceral. Then she shudders and seems to collapse inward, curling over and crying. Not sobbing, not screaming, not flailing at the air or, in her mind, at Uncle Dan. Just weeping, trying all the while to stop herself from feeling anything.

"How long did this go on? Do you remember?"

"Maybe until I was about twelve or thirteen. We moved away at that point. Then I didn't see him much anymore."

We sit in silence. The peaceful room seems like a movie set and Joanna like an actor taking a break from a grueling scene— one that has simply played itself out, requiring the actor's skill and emotional sleight of hand but nevertheless remaining only a parody of a real event. I feel suspended, too. I can't imagine what it was like to be Joanna, that child, that adolescent. I can't imagine what it is like for Joanna now.

"Do you think your parents knew?" I ask.

Joanna shakes her head. "I don't know. Dan was my mother's favorite brother. He was only a year younger than she was. They were almost like twins growing up. Maybe she couldn't believe anything bad about him. Or maybe my father felt indebted to him. For a while, when my father's business was failing, Dan helped us out a lot. Who knows? Maybe they had no idea. That's what I have to tell myself." Joanna looks down and rubs her hands together, as if they were still sticky and in need of washing. "You know, my mother died, and so I can never ask her. I'd like to. I'd like to have a talk with her now and find out what she knew."

When Joanna mentions her mother, she begins to weep again, silently, barely moving. I wonder if Joanna's mother was molested by her favorite brother when they were young. I wonder where the chain of betrayal began and where it will end, as if it were an ugly family heirloom that someone, sometime, has to find the courage to throw away.

"You know what's still the worst thing, the very worst thing?" Joanna asks.

"No," I say.

"That I liked it. That it felt good. That I'd lie on the sofa or on my bed or in the front seat of the car and let him rub me because I loved him and it felt good. How can I accept the fact that I went along with it and never said no, never told my parents?"

"Joanna," I say. I take her shoulders in my hands and we make a lopsided square, me on my stool leaning forward, her sitting straight on her chair. "You were a *child*. You had no say in the matter. When we're children, we take innocent pleasure in our bodies. It feels good to be nursed, it feels good to be held and hugged and kissed and rubbed. You didn't know what he was doing to you, and no adult came along to rescue you. All you knew was that your favorite uncle loved you and wanted to be with you."

"But even later, when we moved away and I was older, if a man didn't respond to me by wanting me, by looking at me or wanting to touch me, I'd think there was something *wrong* with me. That I was ugly. That I was stupid. I mean, for God's sake, when I was only thirteen or fourteen I expected everyone to *want* me."

There is no longer any place, here in this small room, for reason or clinical judgment or medical statistics. I could tell Joanna that of course that's how she responded when she was a child and then a teenager, of course she now felt half repelled by, half desirous of sex, of course she'd had a one-night stand with a man who wanted only her body and made sex feel provocative and clandestine again, as it had with her uncle Dan. We repeat patterns of behavior, even if they cause us pain, because they are familiar. They are all we know, and so, in some odd way, they feel comfortable. They feel like home.

But Joanna can't hear me. She can hear only her own recriminations and self-accusations. Right now, she can't fight back.

"It's OK," I say as I move to her side and put my arm around her. "It's OK," I repeat as she cries into my shoulder, into the crisp starched white of my lab coat collar, as I pat her back and let her mourn and weep, rocking me with the sway of her body. For the next several minutes, she is the girl in the car with dark green seats, the small child jumping up and down on the bed like a windup toy, the young woman who flirted and strutted and blamed herself if men didn't respond. For the next several minutes, I am the mother and father who didn't notice and put an end to the abuse. I am the mother who died too soon, who never heard her daughter's lament and who cannot answer any of her daughter's questions. By revealing her story to me, she also tells them.

Then Joanna becomes a grown-up again, the woman who lies still, as if struck down, during an exam. The woman who loves her boyfriend yet feels sick to her stomach at his touch, who worries that she is frigid, that there is something wrong with her body, who defines herself in terms of events she can't quite recollect. She seems bewildered and, at the same time, grateful for our talk.

I remember that I am not her best friend but her nurse practitioner. I roll back on my stool. I hand her a box of tissues. She takes a deep breath and dabs her eyes, blows her nose. She gathers her things: her shoes, her small black leather bag, her arms and legs and heart. She collects herself.

I help her on with her red jacket, and we stand together. I tell her again that I am here for her, that she can call me whenever she wants. "Please," I say, "take care of yourself." For the third time, I write down the therapists' names and hand the slip of paper to Joanna.

"I guess I know what I have to do," she tells me.

Chapter 28

Renée stands in the corner of the nursery, holding her coat over one arm. Marvin has been in the step-down unit for several days now, a grower baby in crib 4. His original roommates, Ray, Anne, and Rosa, have moved on as well. Ray, the sad puny frog, died a week after Marvin was admitted. Anne is in the step-down unit also, in crib number 1, and Rosa went home at a hefty five pounds. Marvin has done the unimaginable and survived.

Now, whenever I visit, I can tell he's a real baby and not some half human, half prehistoric bird. His hair gets thicker and curlier every day, and he opens his eyes a lot, each eye focusing in a different direction. Renée is also changing. Her blotchy pimples are almost gone. Long sleeves hide the dull blue tattoos that decorate her arms. Only one upside-down "R" is visible on her right hand, below the knucklebone. Her bleached straw hair is covered with a red turban, and her dress is bold, striped red and brown. She smells as if she just finished a cigarette.

We're waiting for Loretta and doing something we never did before, Renée and I: we're having a conversation.

"How are things going for you?" I ask. A week ago, she was discharged to a halfway house. She'd been a model patient in Detox, taking her methadone and attending all her group meetings, so they took a chance and let her go. Now, she's required to hold down a part-time job, show up on time, and stay out of trouble. She visits Marvin every day. Sometimes she takes the bus. When she doesn't have the fare, even if it's snowing, she walks.

"Hey, I'm doing OK. I got part-time work at the mall. Selling shoes." She sticks her foot out at me. Red leather, stacked-up wedge heel, the kind that's torture to walk in.

"Ouch, not for me," I say. Renée laughs.

It's ten in the morning. Loretta called me and asked if I'd come up today too. She said, "I think you'll want to be here when I give Renée the good news." I assume she's going to say that Marvin is out of danger and almost ready to go. Out of the woods.

When Loretta walks in and beckons us over to Marv's crib, Renée asks, "Is everything all right?"

"Everything is great," Loretta says.

Renée nods, draws her lips in, purses them together as if she's trying to blot her lipstick. "So, yeah?"

"Family Services had a meeting with the head of Detox and the supervisory board from your halfway house."

I stay focused on Loretta. Renée looks down at Marvin.

"They said that if you continue to do as well as you're doing, if you stay clean and stay connected with the halfway house, they'll let you take Marvin home." Loretta is excited. She clasps her hands, waiting for the impact of her words to sink in. I can tell that Loretta thinks she just gave Renée the biggest gift of her life.

I don't know if I should cheer along with Loretta or shake my head in disbelief. I picture the Detox meeting, the votes cast by the social workers and psychologists. *If she can keep her nose clean, it means one less baby we have to find a home for. Good foster homes don't grow on trees.*

"They said I can take Marvin home?"

It gets quiet, and Loretta seems disappointed in Renée's response. I feel as though I have to do something.

"Oh, Renée," I say, going over to give her a hug. "That's great. Congratulations."

But her face shutters me out and her eyes become smoky and opaque. I move back and keep my hand lightly on her shoulder.

I'm thinking, *What home? How can they possibly believe that this will work?*

"You're not OK with this?" Loretta asks.

Renée doesn't cry, and she doesn't lower her head.

"Put him in foster care. I don't wanna take him. Not ready, not ready." She shakes her head. "I'm not ready."

Loretta looks as if someone just smacked her in the stomach— half hurt and half angry. "It's your decision, Renée." Renée looks over at Marvin, curled like a shelled shrimp in his plastic house.

"What happens if I don't take him now, but I get him later?"

It occurs to me that Renée has more sense than the psychologists and social workers put together.

Loretta sits down. "I gave up my son when he was born, and he looked for me when he was grown up, about twenty."

"Did he find you?"

"Yes. He called me one day, and we met for coffee."

"Does he love you?"

"He didn't in the beginning. He didn't understand why I gave him up."

"Yeah?"

"But he understood after I explained it to him."

"Why'd you give him up?"

"I was a teenager. I couldn't even take care of myself, let alone take care of a baby. I wanted him to be protected and to have all the opportunities I couldn't give him."

"So does he love you now?"

"Now that we've gotten to know each other. He says he loves me *and* his other mother, the one who raised him."

"I ain't gonna wait that long. Twenty years. I'm gonna get Marvin in a couple of months."

"No matter what, there's a bond that forms between a mother and her baby. That bond's hard to break."

"It's not that I don't *want* him. I want him, I'm just not ready, you know?"

"Renée, what do you mean by 'not ready'?" I ask.

She turns to look at me with her eyes the color of milk and cocoa and her turban dazzling under the bright nursery lights.

"I got things chase me in the middle of the night, you understand? That stuff don't leave you alone. How do I know I won't get up and go out and score, even with Marvin there?"

I see the demons Renée's talking about. They cling to her fingertips and nestle close to her ear. They're transparent as an empty syringe, their voices tinny and sharp.

"But I can't tell Family Services," she says. "What'll they do if I don't take him?"

"I'm not sure," Loretta says. "They'll place him in a foster home. They may ask if you want to sign papers to let him be adopted."

"I don't want him adopted out! I did that for one baby, and I'll never do it again. I said I want him in foster care for *a while*," Renée says. Her voice is loud. It swirls around us, vibrant as the colors in her dress.

Baby up for adoption. What we call BUFA, written in big block letters on the front of a pregnant woman's chart so everyone knows: Don't ask her about the color of the baby's room or the date of the baby shower. Ask her if she wants to hear the baby's heartbeat before you put the fetone to her belly. If she doesn't, go into the back room and get the one with earpieces, like a fancy stethoscope. While you listen, the gallop of the baby's heart pulses directly into your brain and the mother stares up at the ceiling. She tries to ignore the small feet tapping at her insides. *I'm here,* they beat out. *Even if you won't listen.*

"If you want," Loretta says, "I can talk to Family Services. I think if they understand you want to wait for Marvin's sake, they'll go along with temporary placement."

"I'll see him every day, honest. I'll visit just like now," Renée says. "You know, I just can't keep him with me."

This I can understand. I know how darkness elongates the hours and magnifies everything: the sounds, the regrets, the things that go bump in the night and turn you into a child again, no matter your age and no matter how sane you are in the light of day. I, too, have tossed and turned, repeating to myself the litany of the *if onlys*. I can picture Renée holding on, trying to make it until the first hint of dawn creeps under the window shade.

Renée nods. "Yeah," she says. "If you could do that . . ."

So they exchange information, like undercover agents. She gives Loretta the number of the halfway house and the shoe store in the mall. Loretta gives Renée her hospital beeper number and the inside nursery extension. Renée's taking a risk. When *she* thinks she's ready to take Marvin home, Family Services may not agree. If she waits too long, Marvin might be lost in the system, bounced from one foster family to another. But she's right. Taking Marvin home when she's not sure she'll stay clean would be a bigger risk.

"So I gotta go to work now," Renée says and puts on her coat. It's the same deep red as the stripes in her dress, everything threadbare and a size too large. "When are they gonna take him?"

"I don't know, Renée. He's ready to go anytime now," Loretta says.

"I could come back tomorrow and he'd be gone?"

"Well, it probably won't be that soon. I promise I'll call you so you can come in and say good-bye."

Renée stands over Marvin, but she doesn't pick him up, doesn't stroke his cheek, as if it's too painful to have any contact at all. I think if she touches him now, she won't be able to turn away. The three of us wait. Renée doesn't move. Watching her, I remember something that happened between us years ago. She was between pregnancies, between boyfriends, but she'd come in with a raging outbreak of herpes. When I said that she ought to be more careful about the men she slept with, Renée exploded.

"Do you know what it's like to be me?" she asked, jutting her face toward me and accenting her question with one finger, jabbed first at me, then at herself.

"No," I said. "Tell me."

And she did. For thirty minutes, Renée told me her story. The sound of her voice echoed in the room, bounced around in the hallways and out into the world, and I was the world, listening. "You don't know nothin' about me. I got started by my mama when I was ten—men and drugs, sleeping here and there or not sleeping at all. What was you doin' when you was ten? You don't know. You don't know what it's like to live on the street and have nothin'. You don't know what it's like to be me. You oughta try it some time."

Listening to Renée, I realized how many stories are embedded within any woman's narration. I also realized how the layers of a woman's story expand and overlap as we caregivers hear and then retell her words, framed and distorted by our own emotional bias, to social workers and residents who each hear the plot differently and alter it yet again, removing it further and further from the original telling.

I wished I had the multilensed vision of a flying insect, able to see Renée's tale from its many points of view. What if I could know her as her parents did and hear their telling of Renée's history? What if I could know her as a sibling or a neighbor? And now, what if I could be Marvin, relating his version of this woman, this mother?

When I see a patient for the first time and I ask all my myriad questions about how many surgeries and how many hospitalizations, how many cigarettes and who in the family has breast cancer, maybe, to truly understand, I should ask a grief history as well. "How about the tragedies in your life?" I could say. "List for me every unbearable sorrow."

Instead of a pill, the patient and I could then invent rituals to help her across all those painful transitions. What ritual could help Renée now as she leaves Marvin? How will she relocate him in her heart, her mind, her soul?

I imagine her tucking Marvin's things—his newborn cap, the copy of his footprint no bigger than a thumb, the blurry ultrasound picture Eric gave her long ago—into a drawer and, every night, taking them out. I see her pressing Marvin's cap to her face, smelling the sweet new-baby scent. I see her examining the small inked footprint, measuring her hand against it. I see her caressing the glossy ultrasound paper, as if by touching his image she could once again stroke Marvin's soft, delicious skin.

Chapter 29

Being pregnant and giving birth is a normal process, a natural bodily function, not an illness. That's what we tell our patients, particularly the teenagers who come in for their visits moaning and groaning that they can't walk, they can't go to school, they can't help out at home with the chores. They prop themselves up on one arm, rub their bellies. "Oh, my God," they say. "How can I do anything with this in me?"

Sometimes our pregnant teenagers want us to write notes excusing them from school because of harassment. The other kids, they say, tease them or try to push them down the stairs. The stories, like so many we hear in this clinic, make our skin crawl. We get the school authorities and the social worker involved, but too often the schools are no help. It seems they don't really want the pregnant girls around either. "What if they faint?" they ask us. The school nurse asks, "What if they go into labor because they played softball?" Pregnancy is *not* a disability, we reply. No contact sports, no heavy lifting, frequent rest periods, and keep the other kids under control.

School is only one of the problems that Lila, fifteen years old and almost always truant, has at the moment. The biggest crisis looming on her horizon is what will happen when she finally delivers. Meg has already alerted Family Services to evaluate Lila and

Charles's home situation. She doubts that Family Services will take kindly to a baby living in an apartment where the mother is an indentured servant who works for her share of the cocaine.

Lila, it would seem, does her best to perpetuate the problem. She could have moved out to the battered women's shelter. She could have chosen a teen mentor, a woman who would help her through the maze of new feelings, sensations, and responsibilities that constitute pregnancy. She has had access to free at-home tutoring, and by now she could be well on her way to a diploma and maybe a job. But like so many of our pregnant teens, Lila prefers to go her own way. She'd rather be with people she's used to, no matter how they treat her, than with strangers. She'd rather stay in the routine she's accustomed to than venture headlong into an unfamiliar future.

Lila might also have joined the outpatient drug program for pregnant moms and received help kicking her on-again, off-again cocaine habit. But she always insists she is clean, and in truth more than 95 percent of the time her urine screens are negative. When the urine tox does come back positive for cocaine, she says she's mad at Charles and she doesn't care if the baby *is* taken away. Mostly she insists that everything is fine.

———————————

"I'm fine. F-I-N-E, fine," Lila spells out to me as she heaves her bulk onto the exam table. Her cheeks are flushed from today's freezing rain, and she has on a red maternity top that says THIS IS WHAT I'M GETTING IN MY STOCKING FOR CHRISTMAS, with an arrow pointing down to her pregnant belly. I wish Lila's hair were still dyed red, to complete the holiday picture. Her baby is due December 22, and, no longer begging to have the baby removed, she's decided she'd like to go a few days late. She thinks it would be great to have a baby born on Christmas Day.

"I'll name the baby Noelle if that happens," she says. "But Charles still says he wants to name her Angel." She snorts.

While Lila goes on about what a stupid name Angel is, I read the nurse's note, words penned in thick, angry strokes:

Patient not doing her fetal movement counts. Patient complaining of clear fluid leaking from her vagina since yesterday but didn't call. Patient with large bruise on her cheek that she says came from a pillow fight with boyfriend. Patient not willing to meet with nurse educator re: childbirth classes.

The nurse has written down the frustration we all feel. It seems to me that Lila, if possible, becomes more difficult to reach with every visit. As her baby grows, so does Lila's anger. I picture the baby inside and Lila's rage outside, like two big balloons that expand breath by breath until they're about to burst. I get that cringing, ready-for-an-explosion feeling when I look at her.

"So, Lila," I say. "You're due pretty soon. How's the baby?"

She looks down, her favorite evasion. I wonder if she sees something on her knees that I don't. I wonder, too, if she's tired of everyone paying attention to the baby. Lila's the one, after all, whose life stinks at the moment.

"How are *you*, Lila?" I rearrange my face and my mind.

She exhales and leans back on both hands. Her belly is a huge globe riding straight out in front of her. It wobbles and teeters, as if it might be detached and carried somewhere else. When the baby moves, Lila's belly becomes lopsided, then rolls back into position. Her legs are swollen, and her face is doughy. All traces of the spicy red Lila are gone. She has mousy brown hair that matches her mousy brown backpack and her mousy brown life.

"I feel like puke," she answers. In one second, I see Lila's entire life go by, children, old age, illness, death. Quick and sharp, like the crack of a whip.

"I didn't sleep for the past three nights," she says.

Maybe you shouldn't have let yourself get pregnant, I think. Then, *Stop that.*

"I'm sorry, Lila. Tell me about the water leaking from your vagina. What's happening?"

She sits up. "It was just like when I stood up, my pants got wet. I think maybe I peed myself." Lila laughs, a throaty cackle.

I see the bruise by her left eye. It's not old, but not new either. I guess about four days.

"Are you having contractions?" I ask.

"A couple. Like back pain, and sometimes in the front, too. I think it's 'cause me and Charles sleep on the floor since the mattress burned up."

"The mattress burned up?"

"Yeah." She examines her knee. I give her a few seconds; I don't feel like a verbal tug-of-war. Smoking in bed? Cigarettes or crack? Or a match in anger? Maybe Lila tried to torch Charles. Or maybe Lila tried to torch Lila.

"Are you still leaking water today?"

"I don't know."

"We're going to check you. If you're leaking amniotic fluid, we'll want to get you delivered to avoid any infection getting up to the baby."

The royal "we." I can see twelve of us, a team, coming in and pinning Lila down on the exam table. *We're going to do your exam now, my dear.* Here I am in my white coat, my stethoscope over my shoulders, my hands clasped around Lila's manila file with the red sticker on the front indicating "high-risk pregnancy," a yellow dot stuck in the middle of the red for "drug abuse." My mind-camera changes angles, goes to the ceiling. I'm a small white stick figure in the corner. Lila's a mattress glowing red and burning on the end of the table.

"Are *you* gonna do my exam?" she asks.

"Yup." I can't tell if she's happy or planning to bolt before I can lay a hand on her.

"OK, as long as it's you. Do it now, 'cause I got to go."

Given such a generous reception, I hurry to assemble what I need in order to do a sterile speculum exam, what we call a ROM check, to look for evidence that there has been a rupture of the membranes surrounding the baby. Sometimes the bag of fluid doesn't actually break with the big gush of water they show on the soap operas or in the movies, but instead develops a tiny tear that causes some leaking and makes a woman come in complaining of a vague wetness. No matter how small the tear, any avenue through which amniotic fluid can escape is also a pathway for bacteria to enter.

Before doing the vaginal exam, I take a paper tape and measure Lila's abdomen from the top curve of her uterus to the top of her pubic bone. Thirty-seven centimeters. Then I run my hands over her belly, identifying the baby's head, bottom, and back. The baby has moved deeper into Lila's pelvis.

"Getting ready, this kid," I say, looking at Lila's face. She smiles and raises her eyebrows at me, distorting the bruise. The baby's heart is steady and strong when I put the fetone on Lila's belly.

"She sounds good, huh?" Lila asks. She's happy that the baby is a girl. The sister she never had. The mother who threw her out. "Tough like me," she adds.

"Right." I help her up so she can remove her pants for the exam.

"So, tough lady, how'd you get that wallop on your cheek? Nurse's note says that you had a pillow fight."

I move behind the curtain while Lila undresses.

"Oh, it's just Charles, you know."

"Ummm?"

"Charles, he thinks I was maybe fooling around with his friend. His friend's, like, a weirdo. If anything, Charles ought to get on his friend for looking at *me*."

I don't say anything, and Lila pulls open the curtain.

"I'm ready already," she says.

I come around, slide the stirrups out of the table, and help her move down. I sit on my rolling stool, adjust the light, pull on a pair of gloves.

"Lila, the speculum's cold. I'm not wetting it because I want to keep it sterile." Her vaginal walls are swollen and purplish, thick with blood and ready for delivery.

The first thing to look for in a ROM check is fluid pooling in the vaginal vault, evidence of the amniotic fluid leak—and there it is, a little pond brimming over and dripping down the speculum handle. Next, I test the pH of the fluid to see if it's acidic, like normal vaginal mucus, or more alkaline. I dip a sterile swab into the pool and dab the swab on a piece of Nitrazine paper. At once, the paper turns a deep cerulean blue, indicating a pH of more than 6.5, much more alkaline than the usual secretions and almost certainly amniotic fluid. I dip another swab, rub the clear water on a glass slide.

"It must be awfully difficult, Lila, living there with Charles and his friend and that other girl. Especially since you've been elected to do all the work. It doesn't help you get off cocaine, either, if they're always using." I take another swab and do a culture of the vaginal walls, then withdraw the speculum. Lila sits up.

"So?" She looks at me and my assortment of swabs and slides. "Can I go?"

"It looks as though you are leaking amniotic fluid, but I want to take a quick look at this slide to be sure. If you are, we'll admit you to Labor and Delivery."

"What for?"

"To have your baby."

My words hang in the air like a rainbow after an unexpected shower. Then they evaporate, as rainbows do, leaving a shimmer of violet in the air. Lila's face undergoes a metamorphosis. First she looks blank, then a light goes through her eyes, traveling swiftly behind the transparent blue of her pupils. A cloud comes and descends upon her. She looks terrified.

"*Now?*"

"If you've been leaking for a few days, there's a real risk of infection."

Lila is silent, slumped over with her hands on her knees. She seems to be thinking furiously, but she says nothing. I wonder if she's counting how many hours since her last coke use and calculating if she and the baby will be positive on the mandatory tests. Or if she's trying to figure out a way to have this baby without telling Charles, then disappear. I hope it's the latter.

"Do you have questions for me before I go look at this?" I've put on a new pair of gloves and I wave the slide in the air to dry it.

Lila shakes her head no.

———————

The microscope is on a table in the utility room, stuck in the corner by the "clean" and "dirty" sinks. There's a small stool in front of the table and a red plastic box on the wall for used slides. I sit, slip the slide under the metal hooks, turn the lens to low power, and flick a switch under the microscope stage, lighting up the thin band of cells. When I look at the slide, the magnified cells look like small, crushed boxes. As usual, I get lost for a moment in this miniature galaxy with its beautiful crystalline shapes and colors, its strange meandering streams and tiny tumbling life-forms.

The smear on the slide dries quickly, branching into amniotic fluid's characteristic fern pattern, like water on a windshield freezing into ice feathers before your eyes. Lila's membranes are definitely ruptured. Now she'll be admitted, her labor induced. I've always thought Lila herself might rupture someday, finally splitting open from the pressure of her life. Instead, this tiny rent has occurred in the membranes surrounding Lila's girl, as if this baby knows there has to be a way to escape.

Something about this inevitability, the certainty of labor and delivery, appeals to me. It's a process over which we have little control once it begins, so we're relegated to the position of gatekeepers, standing by as labor proceeds. Of course, the doctors might argue that we can start and stop labor, we can intervene when there's a problem, we can pluck out babies in distress, we can open the womb and sew it up again. We have bottles and tubes and oxygen under pressure, we have medicines to fight the bacteria, and, if everything else fails, we have *extreme means,* the mystical machines that help one-pound babies breathe, the crash surgeries we pull off when a new mother's blood won't clot or her uterus turns itself inside out.

Having a baby is a natural process. We tell that to everyone, but I know how it can go wrong. Every time I send a mother upstairs to Labor and Delivery, every time a teenager looks at me and asks if everything's going to be OK, I remember the times something unexpected happened. It's a terrible habit, the imagination of disaster. One I have to break, I tell myself, as I go back to Lila's room.

"Well?" she asks as I sit down again. She looks composed. Actually, she looks as if she's planning to go to the mall.

"That water you've been feeling is amniotic fluid."

"Yeah?"

"That means there's an opening in the membranes around the baby where infection could get in. It's important that you have your baby soon. I'll talk to the chief resident, and we'll send you upstairs to Labor and Delivery."

"Can I go home first?"

"No, Lila. You've probably been ruptured since yesterday, and we're running out of time." Anyway, if I let her go home, she might not come back.

"So what will they do?"

"They'll give you some medicine to make your labor begin."

She looks at me with disbelief. It's that *you-mean-I'm-really-going-to-have-a-baby?* look, as if her pregnancy hadn't been a reality until now in spite of the nausea, the fatigue, the growing abdomen, and the stretch marks. In spite of that moving lump that has a personality even in the uterus, keeping you up at night and liking certain voices, responding to specific songs.

"Charles," Lila says. She looks like a child lost in an amusement park, suddenly missing the adult she came in with.

I tell her that she can call Charles from her room upstairs if she wants to. She can also, I emphasize, tell the nurses if she *doesn't* want to see him. There is the slightest alteration in the angle of her head.

I make the arrangements, call transportation, write in Lila's chart. I tell her that I'll check on her later, in fact I'll come upstairs and visit. I settle Lila into a wheelchair and hand her chart to the young man dressed in white who will whisk her out of the clinic. I wish her good luck, bending over so my cheek presses hers for a moment, and then I hold her hand as the transporter rolls her away. She turns, her belly making it difficult, and looks back at me, her dull hair hanging over her eyes, one eye looking bigger than the other because of the bruise. We hang on to each other until we finally have to let go.

Chapter 30

The operating room is cool and humid. White tiles line the walls, and the floor is tile as well, a soothing grass green. Everything within the room shines: the stainless-steel knobs and cranks on the bed; the IV poles that loom over Eleanor, their plastic bags bursting with saline; the round wheeled buckets and the trays of instruments lined up and ready. Emily, gowned and gloved, stands across the table from Dr. May Gibson, the attending surgeon with whom Emily and Yanna will perform Eleanor's hysterectomy. Yanna stands next to Emily. The scrub nurse, a young man with wire-rimmed glasses, stands on a stool guarding his two instrument trays. He rests his gloved hands on a row of Kelly clamps. The anesthesiologist, busy at Eleanor's head, holds a clear plastic mask tightly over her face and occasionally squeezes an Ambu bag attached to the mask. I stand in the corner. When the operation starts, I'll move a step stool closer and stand behind Yanna, looking over her shoulder into Eleanor's open belly.

I'm here partly from curiosity and partly out of support for Eleanor. She asked, "Will you be there?" I replied that as a nurse practitioner, I don't perform any surgeries other than minor procedures in the clinic, so I rarely get to the operating room except as an occasional observer. But when I mentioned that I had worked as a scrub tech in the OR for a couple of years before I became a nurse, Eleanor grasped my hand. "Couldn't you come and observe my surgery, then, just to help keep an eye on me? You wouldn't faint, would you?" I told Eleanor I'd try to arrange it. I'd loved working in the operating suite. Again and again, stygian images from those OR days show up in my dreams and in my poems: *anesthesia time is a nightmare place, of thin steel hands, white-shrouded face.*

"Breathe deeply, Eleanor," the anesthesiologist says. He removes the mask, tips back Eleanor's chin, and opens her mouth. He inserts a flat silver blade and presses it down against her tongue, then threads a clear tube between her vocal cords and into her trachea. He attaches another tube to this endotracheal tube and tapes it in place, winding the middle of a thin white adhesive strip around the tube and pressing the two ends up alongside Eleanor's nose. He presses the tails of another strip down both sides of her chin. Next he turns the IV valve, and the saline dripping into her vein slows in one line, becomes faster in another. Then he sits back on his high stool behind Eleanor's head and begins rhythmically squeezing the Ambu bag.

"She's ready," he says.

A nurse wearing a surgical mask and gloves comes over to the table and uncovers Eleanor. She lifts one of Eleanor's legs, then the other, bending the knees and putting the soles of her feet together until Eleanor seems to be a dancer doing a plié lying down.

Her body looks chalky under the stark light that hovers over the table like a surprised moon. The flesh of her breasts and thighs is relaxed and spread over her body's edges, accentuating the small crinkles in her skin. Emily, Dr. Gibson, and Yanna each do an internal exam to identify the anatomy of Eleanor's pelvis. Is the uterus tipped forward or back? How large does it seem? And the ovaries? When the three doctors are finished, Emily asks if I want a turn. Examining a patient under anesthesia, she says, is an excellent teaching tool.

When a patient is awake in the clinic, no matter how relaxed she is, the abdominal muscles always contract involuntarily, making it difficult to feel the internal organs. But asleep, the body is totally off guard. The muscles are flaccid, the thick wall between *in here* and *out there* softens, and you can feel the uterus and ovaries precisely. I take gloves from a box on the counter.

First I feel the rubbery cervix, shortened by the cone biopsy, then the firm uterus, slightly enlarged and mobile, riding just under the abdominal wall, then the ovaries, almost too small to palpate, the slippery sensation as they slide over my fingers, all these organs immediate under my fingers, almost as if I were able to reach beneath Eleanor's skin and touch them directly.

I am grateful for this opportunity—never before have I felt the internal organs so clearly defined—yet there is something that feels intrusive about this, all of us examining a patient when she is unaware and will have no recollection. Do caregivers take such liberties casually? As I look about the room, I see only concern on the faces of the surgeons, tension and anticipation reflected in the eyes of the nurse and the surgical technician, vigilance in the protective posture of the anesthesiologist. Their respect for Eleanor is tremendous. Standing back, I remove my gloves.

The nurse preps Eleanor, sloshing first soap, then an antiseptic, Betadine, in a circular pattern over Eleanor's abdomen and up to her breasts. Next, she washes out the vagina with big cotton swabs.

The doctors take sterile towels and open them on Eleanor's body, arranging them to leave a window of flesh stained brown by the Betadine. The small rectangle of skin looks as if it belongs to someone else. Behind the anesthesia screen—the drape hung over a steel frame that separates Eleanor's head and neck from the rest of the operative field—she looks waxen, her mouth distorted by the endotracheal tube. The anesthesiologist has taped her eyelids shut to keep the corneas from drying. Her brown hair is stuffed under a flimsy white surgical hat. Only the rhythmic up-and-down plunge of her chest tells me she's alive.

Dr. Gibson nods to Emily. "Go ahead."

Because Eleanor is a clinic patient, Emily, who has already done about seventy-five hysterectomies in her four years of residency, will do the operation. Dr. Gibson will assist as needed, and Yanna, who's only a junior resident, will hold retractors and learn.

Emily takes the scalpel the scrub tech hands her. As she streaks the knife blade over Eleanor's skin, a moist red line appears and Dr. Gibson blots it.

"Bovie," Emily says, and takes the electrocautery knife to continue cutting; its heat seals any bleeding vessels as it moves through the flesh like a stiletto through a ripe avocado. The yellow fat wall divides, and the muscle layer below gleams white and fibrous. Here and there a few tiny capillaries ooze red, like polka dots.

Emily and Dr. Gibson work, speaking only occasionally, and I stand tiptoe on my footstool behind Yanna, looking into the small pit of the operative field. The scrub tech anticipates each instrument and hands it to Emily before she asks. When they have entered the abdomen totally, he hands one thick steel retractor to Dr. Gibson and the other one to Yanna. They hook the retractors over the edge of Eleanor's open wound and pull. Suddenly the bowel pushes out of the incision, loops of pink cellophane.

The surgeons explore Eleanor's organs. They trace the edge of her liver to make sure there's no cancer studding it, hard clumps that feel like colored glass gems riveted to leather. They check the underside of her diaphragm to be sure there are no rough growths clinging like barnacles under a dock. They slide their fingers up her aorta to feel the long chain of lymph nodes next to it, like knots in a string. They pull the translucent bowel through their fingers the way a woman runs a wet sweater through her hands to strip the water without crushing the wool. Nothing. "Everything is clear," Emily says.

Yanna takes warm, wet gauze packs and tucks the intestines out of the way until the body of the uterus lies exposed. Emily places two large Kellys on the cornua, the junctions of the fallopian tubes and the uterus, and hands the end of one clamp to Yanna. Yanna pulls on this Kelly, retracting the uterus to the right and exposing the round ligament that holds it in place. Emily clamps the ligament, then cuts through it, swift and smooth.

"We're taking the ovaries, right?" Dr. Gibson asks.

"Yeah," Emily says. "We talked it over with her. She's over forty-five and already perimenopausal. Seemed appropriate to take the ovaries too. She agreed."

I note how casually they say this. With the removal of her ovaries, Eleanor will instantly enter menopause. Her hot flashes will begin even before she leaves the hospital. But I know that sparing the ovaries doesn't make sense. We're not sure, at this point, if excising only the uterus and cervix would completely eradicate the cancer. Besides, if the ovaries are left, they, too, could cause trouble down the line, such as annoying cysts or new cancers.

The clock on the wall clicks every time the minute hand jumps ahead, and the second hand sweeps around, timing how long Eleanor is under anesthesia, how long it takes the team to do all the intricate cutting and dissecting necessary to free her uterus and ovaries and remove the cervix that harbors its tiny nest of microscopic cancer cells. Every time Yanna extracts a bloody gauze from the open belly and hands it to the scrub tech, he turns and opens it out on a back table. The circulating nurse walks around every so often and counts them, estimating blood loss. Sometimes the anesthesiologist calls out Eleanor's blood pressure or says "Everything's fine up here." The clock inches and clicks, the second hand hums as it speeds around. Emily peels away the filmy attachments of the bladder and the lower uterine segment.

"Careful here," Dr. Gibson says, and Yanna and I strain to peer in.

"Not much scar tissue. Her only previous surgery was one C-section," Emily says. The scrub tech stretches, and the circulating nurse opens a new pack of sponges, pops them onto the tech's sterile tray. Yanna moves her shoulders around, trying to ease the spasms that develop when you have to pull the retractor with all your strength in order to keep the belly open. If Yanna's grip loosens or her back muscles numb and she lets the retractor slide, Dr. Gibson says, "More retraction, Yanna," and the field expands.

Emily talks out loud, directing herself through the surgery. Occasionally pausing to teach us, she indicates some point of anatomy to Yanna and me.

"OK, I'm ready for the ovaries," she says.

"Put your finger under the infundibulopelvic ligament," Dr. Gibson replies. "And watch out for the ureter." Emily secures the ligament with two clamps, cuts down the middle, ligates the stump with a tie and a suture. She does the same on the other side. Now the ovaries are freed up, still attached to the body of the uterus.

The lights are hot, the air is heavy, and the layers of the OR sterile gown hold in body heat. Emily asks for a wipe, and the circulating nurse reaches up carefully to pat Emily's forehead. When I look around the room, all I see are eyes, our faces hidden by identical green masks. Those of us close to the operative field wear clear plastic goggles, like jet pilots who never leave the ground. It looks as if all those here are huddled in their own private, protective shells, but I know they're a team. They talk quietly, their words falling into Eleanor's body. When there's nothing to say, they speak with their silence.

Emily and Dr. Gibson work close to the uterine vessels, dissecting the tissue away in order to free the uterus from its moorings. The scrub tech hands clamp after clamp, then the scalpel, then more clamps, suture, clamp. Yanna clicks the clamps open with one hand to release them when they're no longer needed, gives them to the tech or leaves them on the sterile towel next to the open wound. Emily makes a careful, precise curved incision over the lower uterine segment.

"Bleeder," Dr. Gibson says, and I see a jet of blood squirt up, spattering Yanna's mask and goggles. The team, used to such occurrences, is unruffled, but my heart accelerates. The scrub tech leans in, hands over gauze and clamps, the cautery. Yanna and Emily bend closer, mopping the blood that suddenly obscures their vision. I glance over at Eleanor's face. The anesthesiologist stands up from his stool, leans over the drape to look at the belly, too, anticipating what he should do next in case there's too much bleeding. He checks Eleanor's blood pressure reading, then he calls it out to reassure the surgeons: "One ten over seventy-four." Eleanor is oblivious, deeply anesthetized; it's as if she has gone away and left her body here for us to operate on. The tape that's crisscrossed over her eyes to keep her corneas from drying out gives her the appearance of a cartoon character, eyes X'd out to indicate loss of consciousness.

For the few moments it takes to control the bleeding, there's a flurry of hands and clamps and the sweep second hand seems to whir around relentlessly. Narrow strips of bloody gauze pile higher on the back table. The circulating nurse counts them again.

Then, slowly, the uterus reappears and the belly is once again clean and moist as the inside of a scraped melon. Emily continues to clamp, incise, and ligate until the cardinal ligaments and the uterosacral ligaments are cut and tied. Emily palpates the lower uterine segment and the vagina where they join.

"All the ligaments are completely incised," she announces. Dr. Gibson nods.

"OK, let's take it out," she says.

Emily asks for a knife. With one stroke she creates an opening into the vagina; then she takes the curved Mayo scissors and cuts across it. She and Yanna shell out the uterus from its lodging and lift it up, a few clamps dangling from it like long heavy earrings.

"Clamps," Dr. Gibson says, and the tech hands four clamps, *bing, bing, bing, bing.* Dr. Gibson and Yanna pick up the edges of the vagina like a tent staked out north, south, east, west.

"One twenty over seventy-eight," the anesthesiologist calls out. Now the abdomen must be resewn, but first everything has to be put back the way it was. The deep end of the vagina, where the cervix used to be, must be stitched closed, and all the stumps of all the ligated ligaments must be checked and double-checked to make sure any bleeding has been controlled.

"How's our patient doing?" Dr. Gibson asks.

"Fine," the anesthesiologist's voice comes back from behind the screen.

The tech begins gathering instruments for the count and tidying his table. It's been an hour and fifty minutes since Emily made the first incision, but it feels as if only a few minutes have gone by. As Yanna begins closing the abdomen, layer after layer, Dr. Gibson turns from the table and strips off her gown and gloves.

"Well, you couldn't ask for a nicer case," she says.

I step off my stool and move to the corner of the room. The tech and the nurse are busy counting sponges and needles and instruments, making sure they have the same number they started with and that none has been lost in the deep pit of the belly. I think of Jonah and the whale.

When Eleanor's incision is stapled tight again, the sterile, otherworldly atmosphere dissolves and the room becomes just another room again, the nurses and the tech intent on cleaning and regrouping for the next case. They have no idea who Eleanor is, but they have seen her exposed and opened, held her blood like rainwater in their gloved hands, watched her drop into time and reemerge. The anesthesiologist pulls the tube from Eleanor's throat and gives her oxygen. She begins to stir, her arms and legs writhing, her hands slowly moving up to her face. She tries to scratch her nose, still itchy from the tape. She mumbles something, and the anesthesiologist says, "Eleanor, wake up now. Surgery's over."

The nurse adjusts the pressurized stockings that wrap around Eleanor's lower extremities, rhythmically squeezing to assist blood flow and prevent clots, and places a sanitary pad between Eleanor's legs. Emily and Yanna step back and peel their gowns and gloves, throw the gowns in a hamper. We all take down our masks to reveal ourselves and the red pressure marks that groove our cheekbones.

One, two, three, we hoist Eleanor's body over to the gurney, and the nurse yanks the heavy green sheets from the OR table. The table looks oddly thin, and the stainless-steel knobs and armrests extend awkwardly into space. Emily and Yanna push Eleanor's stretcher into the hall and down toward the PACU, the post-anesthesia care unit, where another nurse will receive it, roll it into a corner, hook Eleanor up to an oxygen cannula, move her IVs to a different set of stainless-steel poles, reconnect her antiembolic hose, and begin to monitor her recovery.

When I leave the OR, the tech walks out with me for a brief break before his next case, and the nurse goes to the wall phone in the now-empty room. I hear her ask for housekeeping *stat*. In the hallway, a patient in a white gown and gauze cap waits on his stretcher. The doctor next to him asks, "Ever have surgery before?" and their voices breeze by me. The man in the gauze cap looks nervous. For now he is present and fully human; soon he will be, as

Eleanor was, just a vacant sleeping body. No, not sleeping—more like a body suspended, the essence of it taken away somewhere and a husk left behind. When confronted with only the body's shell, the doctors and nurses and scrub techs can go to work. If the real body creeps back in or if the husk looks too alive, it's almost impossible to make that first pass with the knife. There's so much in these stark rooms to be wary of. The man nods under his gauze cap and watches as I walk out of the OR suite on my way back to the clinic.

A few hours later, Eleanor is in her hospital room, a liter of IV fluid, lactated Ringer's solution, dripping noiselessly into her vein. She's only half awake, in and out of a heavy postanesthesia sleep that keeps pulling her down. Then her body rises, muttering, and her eyelids flutter. Her husband, Jeffrey, sits by her side, sometimes reaching up to take her hand and comfort it, sometimes letting his shoulders slump. All the while, he watches her face.

Years ago, when my uterus wouldn't stop bleeding, I had a hysterectomy. I still remember what it was like to wake in the green haze of the recovery room. A nurse floated by laboriously in the gaseous mist. When I saw her and realized where I was, I thought, *I'm alive.* The nurse, seeing me stir, came over. "Do you know where you are?" she asked.

When I was considered sufficiently recovered, they rolled me back to my room and into my bed, and I fell at once into the dreamless cavern where Eleanor now languishes, my family poised at my side just as Jeffrey is at hers. I struggled to the surface only when my pain crescendoed. In the middle of the first postop night, two strong nurses gripped my arms and helped me out of bed for the first time. I straightened my legs, then my belly, then my back. Every inch seemed a miracle. Within a day I was able to watch the Winter Olympic Games, played out in miniature on the tiny TV suspended over my bed. While a snowstorm of epic proportions raged outside my hospital window, I watched the U.S. teams ski the slalom or knock off the competition in the speed skating rink. Every time one of our athletes stood center podium with a gold medal strung around his or her neck while the national anthem filled the arena, I wept slow, silent tears and let them meander down my face. I wasn't in pain; it was just that I felt so *cared for,* when I was used to being the caregiver. A few days before, when I had been admitted for my emergency surgery, a nurse had sat on my bed and taken my hand. "I know you're a nurse," she'd said, "but I'm going to pretend you're not." When she was interrupted momentarily she turned away, but she never let go of my hand. She knew I felt like any other patient—lonely and scared.

Jeffrey's trying hard not to look as if he, too, might cry at any moment. He touches Eleanor's face and smoothes her wiry crazy hair back from her forehead.

At first Jeffrey and I don't speak, sharing the silent bond of those who stand witness. We both know that suffering is a portal. When you walk through it, you have a choice: close your eyes and pretend that nothing touches you, or enter it and go down into its depths.

"Do you think this operation will do it?" he asks me. He doesn't say "will cure her of the cancer."

"Yes," I say, "I think it will." I chance putting my hand on his shoulder for a moment, knowing that people on the edge are often able to hold their emotions in check only until someone is nice to them. A touch on the hand or a kind word, and all the sorrow wells to the surface. Jeffrey doesn't stop stroking Eleanor. Their fingers intertwine, knitting themselves together and apart and together again. Outside, a fierce gust of wind knocks against the hospital window and the large pane rattles slightly.

Eleanor moans. There's a tight row of staples across her abdomen, pinching her, and already her organs have shifted to fill up the tender void left by her uterus. In a few days, she will go home. For several weeks she'll live in the land of the almost-recovered, whose inhabitants are too weak to do any heavy chores or housekeeping and just strong enough to read for hours in the rocking chair by the window. Then, hour by hour, her strength will return. She'll grow restless, at last ready to leave illness behind and close the gate on its seductively quiet rooms and its long days of sleep.

I rouse Eleanor and remind her how to press the button on her

PCA unit, a clever device that allows patients to medicate themselves, numbing the insistent postoperative pain. She fumbles for the button pinned to her johnny coat and finds it, presses the end. There's a melodious *bong,* and the syringe resting in its case at the base of the IV stand moves, millimeter by millimeter, delivering a dose of intravenous morphine. I get a blanket from the closet and give it to Jeffrey. He spreads it over Eleanor, smoothes and tucks it.

"You're both doing fine," I say. "It's time for me to go."

Jeffrey stands and extends his hand to clasp mine.

His hazel eyes have small flecks of gold in them, and his close-cropped gray hair and prominent ears make him look younger than his age. As he talks, he gestures with his hands, as she does.

I leave Jeffrey and Eleanor to sit alone and help each other along. Outside, it's beginning to snow. I wish Eleanor had the Winter Olympics to keep her company.

As I drive away, a million white splotches smack against my windshield and shrink the universe. Unlike all the patients whose lamps shine down from the high hospital windows, I am healthy, wide awake, free to go. So often I have witnessed suffering and marveled at its paradox, how it is both agonizing and beautiful. I have observed how illness contracts a patient's world until only the surgeon's hand, the cool bed, the relief of pain, and the presence of loved ones are important. Once again, standing over Eleanor's body as it was opened and probed during surgery, I have been to the wild, penumbral place and walked away.

At home, still drunk with gratitude for my glimpse into the living body, I greet my husband expansively. Later, getting ready for bed, I run one finger over my own hysterectomy scar, a pink ridge that has almost completely disappeared, faded like the melody of an old Ella Fitzgerald tune—jazzy, hot in its day, and strangely comforting.

Chapter 31

Lila's face is red, her lips dry. Her brown hair is damp and clings to her neck. Every time a contraction comes, she screws up her face and opens her mouth as if she sees something terrifying, but no sound comes out. The TV is on in the corner of the room, and every once in a while Lila hears the sound of muffled laughter. Her contraction increases, sending the baby's heart rate down to a slow, steady thump on the monitor. The contraction graph peaks, and the nurse says, "That's a good one." Then she readjusts the monitor, trying to keep track of the baby's heart. When the contraction ends, the baby's heart rate comes up again, a quick loud booming that competes with the TV's laugh track.

Lila has been in hard labor for hours. When she first arrived on Labor and Delivery, a nurse inserted an IV and drew some blood. She put Lila on the monitor, and when Nina saw the tracing she wasn't happy—the baby wasn't as reactive as she'd like. She did a quick ultrasound and saw that the amniotic fluid level was low, the baby girl curled head down, her fists tucked up by her face.

Nina decided that the baby would indeed be better off outside the uterus than in. She asked the nurse to give Lila some IV Pitocin, medication to start the uterus contracting, and she asked Lila if anyone should be called.

Lila hesitated for a moment. "No," she replied. "No one."

Down in the clinic, shortly after Lila went upstairs, Charles called, asking where she was. Whoever answered the phone told him she was in Labor and Delivery, and a few hours later he arrived. He told the volunteer at the main desk on the first floor that he was Lila's husband. At the entrance to Labor and Delivery, he said the same thing to the ward clerk.

When he walked into Lila's room and found her undressed and in labor, he said, "Why the hell didn't you call me?"

Lila said nothing. Nina asked her if she wanted Charles to be escorted out, but Charles glared at Lila until she said, "No, let him stay." He settled himself on the sofa in front of the TV and hasn't left the room since. He has the remote control in his hand. When Lila begins moaning, he aims the control and punches up the volume.

Nina has been clomping in and out of the room every half hour, her patent leather clogs announcing her arrival. The nurses are afraid of Charles and give him a wide berth, but Nina punches him in the arm and says, "Get over with your girl, man, she's having *your* baby."

These last hours have seemed, to Lila, like a lifetime. In the beginning, the pains weren't too bad, but soon, as the contraction-triggering Pitocin dripped steadily into her vein, she felt a stranger climb into her body and take control. The pains started in her back and peaked in her belly, sending spears of pressure into her thighs. Then, she said, the pain became unbearable. The nurses drew diagrams for her, showing how the cervix shortens and opens, how the baby's head descends into the pelvis. They held up their hands to show her what it meant when Nina said she was three centimeters dilated, then four.

"When you get to ten, the baby's coming," they told Lila, and on the next check, Nina said she was five centimeters, getting there.

Lila's face, the nurses noticed, was wild and disheveled. They brought ice for her lips and cold washrags for her forehead. In the hallway, the nurses cursed Charles for ignoring Lila, watching TV or reading the newspaper instead of encouraging her, and Nina called him a bastard. The next time Nina closed the curtain to check Lila's cervix, Lila caught her arm: "When the baby's born, I don't want his name on the birth certificate, OK?"

Nina said that was fine. And when the baby's born, she added, do you want him to hold her?

"No. I want him out of here," Lila said.

"Should we call Security now?" Nina asked.

Lila thought about this while Nina checked her, then said, "No, I'll tell him when I want to." Nina called Security anyway and put them on alert. She told the nurses, too, and they told the ward clerk. All evening and all night everyone walked around with big eyes and pounding hearts, waiting for Lila to give the word.

It's nine-thirty the next morning when I stop by on my break and poke my head into Lila's room to see how everything's going. I'm hardly in the door when Lila screams, and one of the labor nurses hurries in.

"Oh God, oh God," Lila says, "I have to go to the bathroom," and she tries to swing her leg over the edge of the bed. Her sheets and blankets are bunched up under her, and they're stained here and there with blood and fluid. Every time she has a contraction, a gush of water comes out. Lila accepts this mess, this slightly sharp smell, as status quo. Charles, who slept on the sofa all night, looks up from his TV show as the nurse grabs Lila's arm.

"No, no," the nurse says and pushes Lila back. "Let's check you here." She takes a peek between Lila's legs, her face registering no emotion, no worry, no fear.

"We've got a baby coming," she says and presses the buzzer to alert Nina. The ward clerk calls Security, and two tall boys with brown uniforms and arms like baseball bats come up and stand outside the door. I move over beside Lila, place my hand on her arm in greeting, then step aside to let the labor team do their work. Nina walks in and puts on her gown and gloves.

"Oh God," Lila says, "Oh God, I have to push." She sits up and paws at the bed rails, making tiny noises that are indistinguishable from the TV. Her eyes have taken on that strange quality of light that women's eyes do when labor is strong and bearing down on them, and she seems to focus on something that no one else in the room can see. She's moving in a different time, out of sync with the second hand spinning around the wall clock, with the red blinking light that indicates that the Isolette is warming in the corner, with the rumble and static of the baby's heartbeat on the monitor. The nurse and the doctor are there to protect Lila when she enters this other place. They have to speak to her in loud voices and give clear directions.

"Lie back now, Lila, and pull up your knees," Nina shouts at her.

"Take in a breath with the next contraction," the nurse shouts.

Lila is panting, her lips are drawn back over her teeth, and her face is hot and dripping. When they shout, she opens her eyes briefly, turns her face to the side, and her eyes glow, seeing what Nina and the nurse cannot. She turns her head again and closes her eyes, closing down the light. She takes in a breath and, as Nina and the nurse shout at her again, pushes as hard as she can. She feels the baby coming down from within her, caught now behind her pubic bone, stretching her vagina until it is numb and her thighs shake.

"Ahhhh," she says and takes in air.

"Again," Nina yells at her. "Another breath, close your lips, and push!"

"Now," the nurse commands. "Push push push, push from your bottom, push this baby out!"

Charles has turned away from the TV, one arm extended along the sofa top, one arm resting with the remote control in his lap. He wears dark glasses in this room illuminated by the overhead spot and the one piercing bulb behind Lila's bed. The curtains, heavy and floral, are open behind him, and beyond the curtain is the parking lot, and down the road from the parking lot is the street that leads to Charles's apartment. Although he wrings his hands and occasionally wipes his palms against his legs, he's careful to keep his facial expression impassive, bored.

The baby's head is crowning. Corrugated and malleable, it looks like paper towels sopping wet and crumpled into a ball. Around this damp mass, Lila's vagina is stretched and unrecognizable, a thin lip of pink edging the matted hair and ridged scalp of

Lila's girl. Nina has her hand on the baby's head, exerting just a bit of pressure to keep the baby from coming too fast and tearing the delicate vaginal tissue. Just a touch as the baby's head emerges and the eyes, crunched shut and swollen, and the nose, flattened and translucent, slide into view.

"Here she comes, your baby girl," Nina shouts, knowing that her voice has to find Lila in that other land, traveling miles and light-years to reach her. Nina, who has not yet had a baby, who once asked me what that land was like, frightening or filled with harmony, like her Buddha's celestial garden?

Lila is there, in the magic place, and she has only one purpose now, to bring forth her baby girl. All she knows is that at some imprecise moment in the past months of pregnancy, she has begun to love her baby furiously.

Nina imagines flowing gardens. The nurse studies the light in Lila's eyes, mystified by it as she is at every delivery. Charles sees the shapeless mass that emerges from Lila as it clears and develops eyes, a nose, a mouth, a trembling chin, then turns itself slightly to release a shoulder covered with white paste, another shoulder, a thin, frail chest, and suddenly a tiny whole child with legs that spring open, purple feet that become pink, toenails and fingernails like slivers of his own. The baby sees a blaze of yellow, then the orange sun of the labor room light. Her eyes burn and she closes them tight, flying through the cold air, roughly scrubbed and tickled until she wants to cry, mucus rattling in her airways and sucked out, a red rubber smell, then a transient, overwhelming vertigo, the feeling of being rolled and bound, placed in a tight, warm cocoon within reach of Lila, who holds out both arms and welcomes her.

Holding the baby to her chest, Lila half rises on her elbow and calls for Charles. Her voice echoes in the room, intimidating the TV and shuddering the heavy curtains.

"Charles!" she bellows, and everyone else moves away. Charles ambles over, as if to say "I don't take orders from a woman."

"Get out!" Lila screams, straining her face toward his. Then she begins to cry. In between big gulping sobs she says, "I don't want you here. This is my baby."

The two security guards edge into the room past me. They avert their eyes from Lila's opened body. They watch Charles, and they note who else is in the room and where they stand.

Charles takes a step back from Lila, turns to see the two security guards.

"What the hell do you think you're doing?" he demands, punching the air in her direction. He turns again to look at the guards and then back at Lila.

"I'm telling you, get out! I don't ever want to see you again." Lila's face is shining with sweat and tears, tiny tributaries flowing around her nostrils and off the bottom curve of her lip. Nina looks up from her suturing, and the nurse steps in between Charles and Lila. All present move as if they are players in some waking dream.

One of the guards comes over to Charles, and the other guard circles around to the opposite side of the table. The guards are as tall as Charles, and their brown uniforms and thick shoes give them an air of authority. It looks as though they're not close enough to touch him, but if they stretched out their arms, they'd have him.

"Time to go, buddy," one of them says, and the other says, "Let's go now, without any trouble."

"You can't do this to me," Charles says to Lila. He bobs his head and runs his hand over his hair. He moves from one foot to the other, his big high-top sneakers making a muted, hushing sound.

"Yeah, she can," Nina says, continuing to suture the episiotomy that she'd cut right before Lila's baby was born. "Now get the hell out of here before I have the guards call the cops. You refused to sign the paternity papers, so you don't have any claim here. And Lila's asked you to leave."

One of the nurses, afraid of what will happen, comes over to Lila. "Time to take your daughter to the nursery and clean her up," she says. Lila nods and hands the nurse the small, squirmy mound that is her baby, and her courage grows. Now she knows what it means to be responsible for a life other than her own. She stops crying, pulls back her tears.

"I mean it, Charles," she says. "I don't want no more to do with you."

Charles's anger smolders. He clenches his fists and runs his hand over his hair again, once, twice, hard. He moves from foot to foot, and he punches the air toward Lila, making the guards step closer.

"You bitch," he says to her, "you whore," and he swings his elbows up, sharp, as if to knock even the idea of the guards' arms away. Then he turns and walks out quickly and quietly, passing within a foot of me. He looks straight ahead, and I move aside. The guards follow, four paces behind, and one of the guards activates his walkie-talkie. It makes a high-pitched squeak and then a long crackle as they go out of the room behind Charles, into the hall and out through the sliding glass door to the corridor that leads to the elevator.

Inside the room, it's as if nothing happened. Lila lies back, exhausted, and the nurse brings her a cold washcloth. Nina's almost finished with her sewing. She looks up at me and arches her eyebrow.

"Come congratulate your pal," she says. "She just did a great job here."

I walk over and take Lila's hand, and she grabs on tight.

Chapter 32

As difficult as it might be for patients to believe, the details of their bodies fade from my memory almost as quickly as the patients dress and walk out the door. Even when I've seen a patient repeatedly over a span of months or years, I don't remember the exact anatomy of her breasts, the specifics of her flesh, the characteristics of her genitalia. Her nakedness vanishes like a photograph being un-developed. The image that is sharp and clear at the time of the exam disintegrates into a wavering negative and a few lines written in her chart.

I've come to realize that when I look at a patient's body, I inspect it with a kind of double vision. Of course I see the body as it is, but at the same time my eyes scan quickly, drawn only to the details that might signify trouble. *Look here,* my brain directs, *now there, and there.* It murmurs *normal, normal,* then suddenly the room flares as if a beam were directing me, pinpointing the spot where *abnormal* lurks. All the while, the patient and I continue our small talk. My hands move over her flesh as I picture the organs beneath with a focused, depersonalized stare. This way of looking is nothing like my usual eyesight. Although I never approach a patient expecting to find anything threatening, anything out of the ordinary, this special vision is reliable. Like a well-trained, silent sentinel, it appears only when needed, turning itself off and on automatically—although I'm sure this clinical gaze has taken me years to learn.

When I finish the exam, the patient and I sit together and review the only images I will retain. "I saw a mole on your back that I'm concerned about," I say as I picture again the firm black lesion. Or I remember the ulcerated area I saw on her cervix, like a tiny moon crater, and say, "When I was doing your Pap test, I noticed something."

What I recall more often is the rise and fall of a woman's narrative and how I witness the peak and resolution of her anguish or share her moments of delight. Women reveal more with their words than with their nakedness, and it's a woman's words that change me. But I can't recall her body until I examine her again, my fingers and my stethoscope retracing the geography of her flesh like a blind woman might outline once more the shape of a familiar but invisible face. Then story and flesh come together again, and the exam room is transformed.

"Joanna," I say, closing the door behind me, "I haven't seen you in a long time."

Her hair still falls in its precise layers. Her demeanor is still half polite, half reticent, but I notice at once that she seems more *adult* tonight, as if she has left behind the part of her that was the anxious, barely contained child.

"Hi," she says and smiles. Something else. Greeting her, I feel at ease. The air feels calm. The high tension that crackled about Joanna in her previous visits is gone.

"How are you?" I ask, taking the hand she offers. As soon as our fingers touch, the memory of her childhood ordeal floods over me. For a moment I feel disoriented, a little faint. I had forgotten the enormity of it.

"I'm better, I think. I finally called one of the therapists, and she's wonderful. David and I both see her, and I see her alone once a week," Joanna says. Her voice is hushed with gratitude and relief. "It's a start."

"Good," I say. "I'm really glad."

Joanna made this appointment for her Pap test, a simple, routine visit. I'm happy she's returned, yet I know that, for me, there may or may not be any resolution of the conversation we began in our initial meetings. We may or may not recapture the closeness we shared before, when she confided in me for the first time. The clinic, I have learned, is not like a novel in which a tidy beginning, middle, and end give shape and consistency to a story. Women come into my world and, just as quickly, they go. A woman might reveal, as Joanna did, her most intimate secrets. Then her follow-up appointment might be broken or forgotten. The woman might change insurance companies and go to another provider. She might move to another state or simply move on, and so I never learn the outcome of our encounter.

In the next room, another woman will be waiting. She, too, will have her tale, and we will have our hour together. What one patient begins, I have found, is often continued in the text of the next patient's conversation. Nevertheless, in some ways I'm always mourning—the last visit, the terrible diagnosis, the patient lost to follow-up, the lack of closure. Wouldn't my life be easier, I sometimes think, if I could check off patients' problems like a list of chores at last completed?

Yet in other ways, I like this open-ended dialogue. I have come to accept the tension of not knowing. It makes all outcomes possible, and it makes my time in the clinic seem cyclic rather than linear, a pattern as rhythmic as our hormones and as perfect.

Tonight I'm curious about how Joanna feels, how any woman feels, as she returns to face me once again when I have been the one who watched her initial, raw unfolding. Do some patients resent me because now I share their secrets? Are they embarrassed, feeling as exposed and transparent as a child whose parent, like a clairvoyant, speaks aloud the words that child is thinking? Sometimes, when a woman has told me what she has never confessed to anyone, she and I develop a special bond—not friendship exactly, but something more difficult to define. A lasting partnership, as if we have traveled a long way together to a dangerous place, and returned.

Other times, I meet a woman in the midst of a crisis and remain suspended there. At her next visit, I find we cannot step back into the rarefied atmosphere of that initial, heightened sensibility. For a moment, I feel as if I have been abandoned in the middle of the journey we agreed to share. Then I realize that circumstances have changed and I must redefine who she is and what our relationship is, framed no longer by her crisis but by her strength. Patients create new lives in the months and years we are apart.

But Joanna seems to feel the same urge that I do to give our dialogue shape. "I *am* due for my Pap test, but I wanted to thank you, too," she says. "I'd never told anyone before about what happened to me. It was funny. The more we talked, the more I remembered. The more I felt that what happened to me wasn't so—well, so much my fault." Once again, she extends her hand. When I move closer, we decide instead to hug.

As I examine Joanna, we talk about her artwork and about David's new car and our snowy winter. When I do Joanna's Pap test, she says how much she liked the last movie they saw and how she has to take an early train into New York to visit a gallery that might hire her to design its catalogue. I notice that she still lies quietly when I examine her, but not in quite the same doll-like manner. When I open the speculum, she flinches. She says, "We talk about this in therapy. How our bodies hold memories."

After the exam, she asks me if I ever got around to writing my paragraph about who she was. "You know," she says, "based on my list of words?" She sits up and leans forward.

In fact, I looked again at Joanna's words not long after she had given them to me. In between patients, not knowing if I would ever see her again, I scribbled my impression of the woman I thought those words might represent:

> *Light words and somber words. Some words of exposure, others that hide. There is much of the physical here, words with flavor and heft and movement, like raspberry, lemon, sun, swim, shout, painter, and canvas, as well as words that live in the spirit and the recesses of the mind: soul, forget. At one glance, this might be a woman in a still life, captured on canvas by a painter who seems to have an intense longing for revelation.*

But there's also a cry here, some event burrowed into the subconscious, waiting. The words are lined up in exact columns, giving the illusion of control, and yet the words themselves, like prisoners, struggle to break free. The handwriting makes the words weightless, as if they might fly away, but sound and sense bind them firmly to the page. What could release them? What might encourage her to speak these words aloud?

When I'd finished writing, I'd folded the paper and put it in the back room in my locked drawer, the place where I keep my pocketbook, my prescription pads, and all the articles I plan to read. Now I go and take the paper out, unfold it, and hand it to Joanna. I don't know all the answers and I can't always help my patients negotiate the difficult turns or the hazardous cliffs, but I try. Trying to help is trying to love.

She reads, and then she nods, weeping, no longer ashamed to let me see her cry.

Chapter 33

"I'm so confused," Eleanor says with a large grin and a small grimace as she lifts herself onto the exam table. She sits carefully, favoring her incision. The healing scar across her abdomen may still be painful, but her mood is cheerful. The pathology report from her hysterectomy was excellent: no evidence of cancer beyond the cervix; all margins clear; no vascular invasion.

Eleanor and Jeffrey were elated at this news. Suddenly the vague uncertainty of the coming years had lifted, as a morning haze burns off in the afternoon. Once again, Eleanor could talk about the future. She wants, she says, to be as healthy as she can for as long as possible. That's why she's here today. "To settle the question of menopause once and for all," she says, shaking her finger at me. "To know the direction I should take."

Now that it's over, now that she has weathered the tests, the procedures, the surgery, and the early weeks of recovery, I imagine Eleanor must be at her most vulnerable. She has had time to rest and think, time to say to herself "I had cancer." Now all she has to do is find the best way to live the rest of her life. How, she wants to know, can she juggle the many issues and make the right decisions? Hormone replacement, exercise, diet, risk of breast cancer, vitamins, cholesterol, calcium, heart disease, mammograms, bone

loss—she wants answers. I wonder if I should tell her that I'm per-
plexed, too. I also want to find the right formula for a long lifetime.
I, too, want my days to extend beyond the too-brief space of years
bracketed between the parentheses of menarche and menopause,
and I want those days to be healthy, productive, and balanced.

Menarche. We awake one morning or come home from school
one afternoon to discover that a woman has moved into our little-
girl bodies. This new person bleeds, leaving a rusty brown smudge
on our underpants. We try to wash it out like a guilty deed we must
hide from the world, but the red stain doesn't scrub away so easily.
Soon we become accustomed to shedding our blood monthly, a
thick garnet secretion with an odd, warmly pleasant odor we notice and worry about and, in some ways, grow to love. It is magical,
this regular message from our bodies' internal processes, and it
hints at some potential or power we cannot, in adolescence, define.
The regular return of our menses demonstrates that our lives have
rhythm and pattern. This rhythm teaches us that we must pay attention to our bodies; that, in fact, we couldn't ignore them even if
we wanted to.

We also learn to accommodate this intruder's changing form.
Her breasts, puffy at first, then firm and cone-shaped, become
ours. We grow obsessed with her silhouette, looking at ourselves in
the bathroom mirror, turning this way and that, leaning over to see
how far our breasts hang from our chest walls. Sometimes we find
these breasts hateful and wish we could bind our chests flat again.
Sometimes we want everyone to see them. Body hair sprouts where
we never expected to find any, and we become tongue-tied, grace-
less where we were once self-assured. The conversion is complete
when this person enters us totally, *her* moody bursts of anger directed at *our* mothers, her tearful recriminations evolving into our
own adolescent suffering.

In time we adjust. Our hips round and grow, our thighs and
our breasts are delightful or they are not, and we become friends
with our puzzling and ever-insistent bodies. We try hard to accept
ourselves as we are. We think we will never grow old.

Then, when at last we have made peace with these bodies that bleed and desire and transform themselves in syncopated monthly cycles, they change again. This time it feels not as if we are being invaded, but as if we are being abandoned.

Menopause. The someone who moved in so many years ago moves out. Stepping lightly from between the sprung bones of our rib cages, lifting her feet so as not to trip on our ankles, she steals away. We cross off the days, yet there are no more red stains. If there is blood, it has a mind of its own and becomes unmanageable. We bleed through our skirts. Sometimes we pass clots the size of a fist, and when we tell our doctors, they say, "Really?"

When that vagabond woman leaves us, we discover she doesn't go empty-handed. She pocks our thighs and wrings out our bellies. She thins our eyebrows and grays our pubic hair. All night we miss her, tossing and fretting in a vapor of internal heat. Her worst mischief is invisible: she hardens our arteries and softens our bones.

Again, we acclimate. What we had, we let go of. What we want, we must now reach out and grasp. Some of us, like Eleanor, fight illness and win. Many more of us lie awake in bed wondering what our futures will bring. "That's the thing," Eleanor says to me now. "I have to figure out how to get rid of these symptoms."

If only, I think, it were that simple. Technically, it's easy to define menopause: the natural cessation of menstruation, the total absence of vaginal bleeding for one year. This expected change occurs when the ovaries stop producing estrogen and progesterone, ending the menstrual cycles for good. During the months or even years before menopause, a woman's estrogen level fluctuates. This perimenopausal time can begin even in a woman's mid-thirties. She may experience irregular menstruation, heavier or lighter bleeding, clots, and, as Eleanor did, other symptoms as well: changes in sleep and mood, headaches, forgetfulness, anxiety, and a host of other, individualized disturbances.

Sometimes, menopause comes slowly and gently. Other times it drags itself in screaming and hollering. Most women enter menopause around the age of fifty-one, others later, some earlier. Usually we go through menopause at about the same time our mothers did. To some women, like Eleanor and me, menopause arrives swiftly, carried in on a surgeon's scalpel. When the ovaries are removed, hormone production stops abruptly and a woman is thrust into menopause. But no matter how we get there, we're not alone. At the present time, more than thirty-one million women in the United States have experienced the onset of menopause and the end of their reproductive years.

For some, this is a dread event. Menopause holds a mirror up to our society's fears: the loss of supple youth, the worry that our sexuality may wane, the visceral understanding that superficial beauty is indeed transient. For others, menopause is part of a natural cycle, not an illness but a process as inevitable as birth, aging, and death. In the clinic, it's mostly the North Americans who view menopause as an enemy. My other patients seem to hold a worldview in which menopause is simply a part of their difficult lives, in which only poverty, illness, hardship, and war—not routine bodily changes—are counted as problems.

———————

"When I was growing up," Eleanor says, "my mother never mentioned menopause. She told me all about menstruation and how babies are made, but she never mentioned *this*." She sweeps her hands down over her torso, suggesting, perhaps, that she had been unprepared for the changes her body would undergo. What she says is true: menopause is the big mystery. Mothers and daughters rarely discuss this stage of the reproductive years, and if we do, we focus on the symptoms, the flushes and sweats and moodiness. What we should talk about is how to prevent what might happen over the long run: heart disease and osteoporosis. We should also talk about how this body alteration might give us the opportunity, happily, to rearrange our lives. In the hiatus that occurs between middle and old age we might find more time to ponder, to create, to extend ourselves to others.

"So," Eleanor says, "here are my questions. If I take estrogen to end these bloody hot flashes and help my bones, am I going to get breast cancer? And how much calcium am I supposed to take?

Good Lord, I can see myself lining up my pills every morning." As she bemoans her plight, she laughs her hardy laugh. When you've been released from death, after all, everything else becomes minor.

"If I knew what we should do, exactly, to keep ourselves healthy, Eleanor, I'd tell you," I say. "I can only give you the advice of the moment. Who knows what they'll say ten years from now?"

I tell her about the old medical books I collect, how I read them now and smile at the outdated "knowledge." In one book from the 1950s, a physician author states that the severity of menopausal symptoms varies tremendously with the "emotional stability" of the individual woman. "Crying and general irritability, particularly toward members of her immediate family" appears second on his symptom roster, and his first option for management of menopause is psychotherapy. The second is occupational therapy: "Any job, project, or interest which focuses the patient's attention away from herself will be of benefit." As a backup treatment he suggests a sedative, elixir of phenobarbital, four cubic centimeters every four hours with larger doses for "cases of frank hysteria."

"The scary thing," I say, "is that back then, this was gospel."

Eleanor and I both laugh, but our laughter is hollow. We look at each other, and what our eyes say is "And what we believe today may turn out to be wrong as well. How can anyone be sure?"

"I suppose I'm most worried about breast cancer," she says. "I read some report where they found that if you take hormones, your risk increases."

I read that report too. In fact, I've read hundreds. Breast cancer *isn't* our biggest threat, but it's the most disconcerting. But all I have to offer Eleanor is a scattering of "facts," some that might prove true over time, others that might not. I tell her that if postmenopausal women on estrogen do develop breast cancer, it's usually detected sooner. I say it's also more likely to be a type of cancer that's slow-growing and therefore more treatable.

"Keep in mind that more women will develop heart disease than breast cancer," I say. "It's best if women look at their own individual risk factors before making a decision about taking estrogen."

"Let's do that," she says, folding her hands in her lap.

"Remind me," I say. "Do you have a family history of breast cancer?"

"No."

If she had said yes, I would have told her about the advances in genetic screening and how she might be tested, but I'd also have told her that most patients who get breast cancer have no risk factors other than their advancing age. If she had close relatives—a mother, aunt, or sister—with breast cancer, I'd encourage her to think carefully about hormone therapy, and I'd try to help her decide if, for her, the benefits outweighed the dangers.

"In any event," I say, "I think women should be vigilant. We should examine our breasts, let a professional examine them at least annually, and I believe that yearly mammograms do help detect breast cancers early."

I don't mention that I had that run-in with suspicious microcalcifications and so I'm more cautious. I don't say that for a while I'll be repeating my mammogram every six months or that I cut my own estrogen dose in half.

"So I'll have a mammogram every year," she says. "Now, what about my bones? Am I going to be an old stooped-over lady like my grandmother? She had quite a dowager's hump." Eleanor hunches over and mimics her grandma's bent-over posture.

When she does, I think of my mother, who, like Eleanor's grandmother, was frail and stooped as she walked, her bones as delicate as a sparrow's. I remember my mother falling. First it was her wrist, broken when she slipped on the icy patio on her way to fill the bird feeder. Then it was her hip, fractured as she tumbled from a nursing home bed.

Even as I recall my mother, seeing the image of her body lost in the huge white expanse of the hospital bed, I'm trying to formulate what I will say next to Eleanor. At the same time, I'm thinking how wonderfully layered my interactions with patients can be—how easily, in the midst of a clinical discussion, I can be rocked by personal memories or feelings. I have no doubt that this happens to my patients as well. While I'm rambling on about some test or bit of information, they might be elsewhere, lost in dreams or despairs that have been evoked by a single word.

Today, perhaps because we're addressing issues of aging, I'm feeling somewhat melancholy. Eleanor, too, seems not quite herself but more brusque—as if she has something else on her mind but, like me, must first attend to the business at hand.

"Anyway," I say, "just being a woman increases your chances of osteoporosis. Other risk factors include having a family history, smoking, alcohol, being postmenopausal, having a slender build . . ."

Eleanor's laughter interrupts me. She roars, throwing back her head. "Well, I qualify on family history, but I don't think you could call me slender anymore." She wipes her eyes, and I think how much I love it when laughter brings tears. Our sorrows and our joys, balanced so precariously.

As we go on talking, I try to be professional and complete, addressing all the myriad issues of menopause, and Eleanor either hurries me along or else she jokes, stopping the clinical flow and asking me about my own health care decisions and what *I've* decided to do as I age. Sometimes I tell patients my personal business and sometimes I don't. Today, because it's Eleanor, I answer her questions.

When I recommend regular exercise and calcium as ways of combating the loss of bone mass that runs in both our families, Eleanor asks me if I exercise.

"I try," I say. Most nights after work I put on my sneakers and go into the basement, where our ten-year-old NordicTrack awaits me. I turn on the TV and crank up the leg tension, and off I go, twenty minutes to make my heart pound and my arms and legs ache. I like the way it feels, the movement of bone and muscle and skin.

When we talk about hormone replacement, she asks, "Do you take it?"

"I wear an estrogen patch," I say. "A small dose in a patch I stick on my skin and change once a week." Then we talk about whether or not Eleanor might want to consider using estrogen replacement therapy herself, taking a pill every day or wearing a patch.

Somewhere during our conversation, in our exchange of anecdotes and information, it occurs to me that we are creating a portrait: the two of us, together here in exam room 6. It's a picture I will hold in my mind's eye.

"Look at us," I say. "Two ladies sitting here and talking. So many decisions."

For the first time, she fidgets and looks unhappy.

"What are you thinking?" I ask her.

"It just seems like so much to *do*. Take calcium, get your mammograms, don't drink or smoke, eat right, take estrogen and then worry about breast cancer or else don't take estrogen and worry about breaking your hip while you're exercising. Walk out the door and get run over by a bus."

"I know," I say. "It seems overwhelming. We can only control what we're able to control. Not smoking. Exercising. Maybe using hormones, maybe not. But we can't do anything about that bus."

"I'll have to do some thinking," she says. "I have to decide if I want to take estrogen, and then I have to decide if I should lift weights or take up hiking. I may have to retire just to find time to keep myself going."

"You've already got the most important ingredient of a successful menopause," I say. "A good sense of humor."

The next thing Eleanor says takes me totally by surprise.

"No," she says. "The most important ingredient is a good caregiver. And, unfortunately, I have to find a new one."

I look up at her. I realize, all at once, that Eleanor has really come here today to say good-bye.

"Jeffrey has found, thank goodness, a new job. But in two weeks, I'll be covered under his health insurance, and then, they tell me, I can no longer come to the clinic. I have to find a private doctor in the community." The creases around her eyes and mouth deepen. Her crazy hair is loose today, a trembling scribble of brown around her handsome face.

"I'm going to miss you," she says. "You've all been wonderful to me."

For a moment I'm silent, aware of a hollowness in my stomach, a vacancy in my chest. A favorite patient is moving on. Part of my sorrow is personal. I've grown close to Eleanor, and I like her very much. Part of my sorrow is professional as well. What will happen to her over the years? Will she be healthy, or will her cancer recur? While our final farewell may lend some emotional closure to the months I have known Eleanor, it will be, as well, a harbinger of uncertainty. Her clinical course will remain forever unknown to me. A closed door. An unfinished puzzle.

"Oh, Eleanor," I say. "I'm glad to hear about Jeffrey's new job, but I'm sad that you'll be leaving. I've enjoyed knowing you so much. I'm going to miss you, too."

"Well," she says, "we've been through a lot. So let's not say good-bye. Just give me some information to read about estrogen, and I'll call you in a few days with my decision. And I've got to come back to pick up my records. Maybe you'll never get rid of me."

Holding her hand against her belly, she gets off the exam table. "Damn incision," she says. "It pinches, but I pretend it belongs to someone else."

Good, I think. Eleanor's not going to let anything hold her down.

I give her some pamphlets about hormone replacement, and I tell her to call if she decides she'd like to use estrogen. I add that she could also wait and discuss this again with her new caregiver.

"No," she says, grinning. "You'll do."

"Is there anything else I can help you with?" I ask. There is no easy way to end a relationship with a patient.

Eleanor smiles. "Just answer one last question. Will I live to be a cantankerous old lady?"

"Without a doubt," I say.

Eleanor puts on her coat and wraps a scarf around her neck, prepared for the cold wind that appeared earlier today, threatening more snow. As we head out toward the desk, she slips her arm over my shoulders, a warm, slightly uncharacteristic display that I accept with pleasure.

She squeezes my shoulders.

"We'll be fine," she says. "It's just another phase in the grand adventure."

Chapter 34

Lila decided, after all, to name her baby Angel. It's been six weeks since Angel was born on a Tuesday, the second week of December. Six weeks since Lila has had a cigarette or been threatened by a man. In the clinic, our patients come in with slush on their boot soles and layers and layers of clothing. To measure a girl's pregnant belly, I have to peel back corduroy pants, long underwear, fuzzy tights, and finally the limp elastic of worn-out cotton underwear. Underneath, the stretched-tight skin is rashy and chapped.

Angel is wrapped in a pale yellow blanket and stuffed into an infant carrier. Under the blanket, she wears a one-piece snowsuit and a big-brimmed cap. Under the cap, a pink headband circles her forehead, a fabric rose right in the middle. She has new-baby navy blue eyes, tea-colored skin, and brown hair that wisps over her perfect ears. We see lots of babies here in the clinic, and *this,* we say to each other as we gather around Lila and Angel in the hallway, is a beautiful baby.

I take off Angel's cap, and the nurses and residents and I exclaim over the shape of her head, the curve of her cheek, the long eyelashes that Lila insists come from *her* side of the family. Angel sleeps deeply as we tickle her chin and lift her tiny hands, hoping she'll curl her fingers around ours. We gently cup her head, asking if she remembers a time before she was born. The nurses congratulate Lila, and Lila tells them her version of labor and delivery, how Nina delivered the baby just in time, how she herself threw Charles out as if he were so much trash. Girls in the waiting room, newly pregnant, lean closer to listen.

When her tale is finished, Lila looks over at me and says, "I hope I'm gonna see *you* today."

I'm pleased that she asked for me when Yanna is her favorite resident and Nina delivered her. It's a new year, and maybe this is a new Lila. I admit, I half expected to see Charles arrive with her today. Too often, our patients escape bad relationships just to show up with the same partner a few months later. Absence dulls their bad memories, and they find it difficult to live alone without money or an occasional good time. Sometimes, a woman figures the trouble she already knows is better than the trouble she hasn't met.

Claire guides Lila to room 5. I wait outside in the hall, leaning against the map with its pearl-headed pins that trace the wide arc from North to South America. Claire takes forever asking Lila the usual postdelivery questions and doing her intake: weight, blood pressure, urine dip. I return a few phone calls, see a quick pregnancy visit, and wander around waiting for Claire to tell me that Lila's ready for her postpartum exam. The exam is easy. It's the talking part that's hard. *How are you doing, you and the baby? Do you have enough money and food? And are you safe from the boyfriend who hit you?*

How about a girl who just turned sixteen? How do you help this girl and her baby survive? No, more than that. How do you help them to flourish? Claire hands me Lila's chart.

"Put on your seat belt," she says. "She's a jabbermouth today."

Lila sits sideways on the table. She has placed Angel, still in her infant seat, on the floor next to her. Lila has lost weight. She's almost as skinny as she was at her first visit, with ribs like ladder rungs and shoulder blades that stick out like fins. She has no belly anymore. The lump that was Angel is gone, leaving only a few stretch marks, silvery as fish scales, as evidence. Lila has undressed and put on the cloth top, open in the front as she was instructed. She left the lap drape folded up, a small white square balanced on her thighs. She's wearing her gold hoop earrings, the ones that spell "Lila" along the edge. Her hair is red again, recently cut. I take the drape and open it over her legs.

"Hey hey!" Lila greets me, making me laugh.

"Lila," I say. "It's so good to see you."

It's warm in the room, and I hear Angel's harsh breathing.

"How about I open Angel's snowsuit and give her some air?" I bend to loosen the blanket, unzip the suit, and pull Angel's arms free.

Lila jitters her leg up and down, making her earrings dance. Her fingernails are chewed down, the cuticles jagged as the rickrack my mother used to sew on my skirts when I was seven. Lila has nail polish on. As I fuss over Angel, Lila jumps down to attend her, moving my hands away as new mothers often do. A good sign.

While she finishes unwrapping Angel, she begins to chatter again about her labor: the hours in pain, the way Nina and the nurse ignored her and let her split open, *finally* pulling the baby out.

I sit on the stool and look at her. I guess Lila wanted to see me today because I was there. I've been a part of her grand adventure all along.

"I got an apartment," she says, climbing back onto the exam table.

"Great! Tell me about it."

"I got this friend named Charlene. She was gettin' the apartment and wanted a roommate, so she said I should move in," Lila says.

"What's the apartment like?"

"You know where Stop & Shop is? It's the building right beside the parking lot."

Lila draws pictures in the air and describes the apartment. One big window with a view of the store. Another small window in the bathroom that overlooks the swampy land behind the building where cattails wave and rattle in the cold wind. The one-year lease is in Charlene's name. "So Charles," she whispers, "can't find me." I picture Lila looking out the window at the shoppers, their arms overflowing with grocery bags.

"Lila," I exclaim, "I'm *really* happy to see you're doing so well."

She squirms and flips her earring around. "Isn't Angel *adorable?*" she gushes, looking down at her baby.

Angel, born on a Tuesday and therefore filled with grace. I'm glad to see that she's clean and dressed in all her finery. I think of the stories in the newspapers and on the radio. I remember all the children who were abandoned or simply allowed to drift away, emotionally or physically. The street kids, like Lila. Where will she and Angel be in twelve years? *Who* will they be?

Lila laughs at the way the sheet keeps slipping and tickling her. She crumples it and sticks it under her thigh. Then, like a little kid, she bats at the johnny coat's sleeves, floppy and too big for her skinny arms. When she calms down, she asks if the cat got my tongue.

"I'm wondering how you are."

"Are you kidding?" Lila purses her lips. "I'm fine." She stops fidgeting and seems to swell with pride. "Angel sleeps through the night every night."

"Wow," I reply. "Lucky for you."

Lila stares at me. Her foot goes up and down, up and down.

"So do the exam already," she says, and I can see her trying to put a lid on, trying to still the energy. In the corner of my mind, I wonder if Lila's jumpy because she's using.

"I owe you an apology, Lila. You were trying so hard during your pregnancy to stay away from drugs, and I didn't realize what a good job you were doing. How's it going now?"

She looks right at me, angry that I'd even ask. "I'm *not* using," she says. "I have a baby to take care of."

"Good. How about Charles? I hope he hasn't found you." *I hope you haven't told him where you are.*

"Oh," she says. "Well, I seen him once downtown, but he don't know where we live." Lila looks at me and laughs, makes a raspberry noise. "Look at your face," she says. "Don't *worry,* I'm not stupid."

After Angel was born, Lila stayed in the hospital two days. She didn't have a car seat, so the social worker obtained one from a local agency along with some used baby clothes. The day Angel and Lila were discharged from the hospital, Nina and I followed them into the lobby and watched as they negotiated the automatic doors that opened with a suck and blast of cold air. Before she got into the taxi, Lila put down the infant carrier for a moment and bent to adjust Angel's cap and snuggle the blankets around her, a gesture that all mothers everywhere know—that quick tug, that last check to make sure their child is warm enough, protected. She secured Angel in her car seat and slipped in next to it, gesturing to the cabby with one hand, patting Angel with the other. Nina and I hugged our lab coats around us and waved. From where we stood, Lila looked like a young woman instructing the world where she wanted to go and exactly how she planned to get there.

That's the image of Lila that I choose to hold in my mind's eye.

"So what do you want from me?" she asks.

I laugh. I know Lila's not talking philosophy, but I say, "I want you to have a good life."

"Yeah? What's your idea of a good life?"

Good question.

"Being healthy. Having food and a place to live. Coming and going as you please. Working or going to school. Being able to love your kids and give them a chance. Having some fun once in a while. I guess there's a lot to having a good life."

"Easy for you, being rich."

"If I were rich, I'd be home eating chocolates."

Lila snorts. "Ha ha. Real funny."

"Does Charlene give you a hand with Angel?"

"Sort of. She can't change a diaper very good."

"And you have enough money for food and clothing?"

"Yeah, yeah." Lila has a bemused expression on her face.

"What?" I say to her.

"You're *so* worried! I'm, like, *fine*."

"OK," I say. "You win. I'll stop talking and do the exam."

"God, finally." Lila slides into position. First I check her breasts. They're flabby, as breasts can be after a delivery, and streaked with stretch marks.

"Would you look at them?" she says. "They, like, deflated when I stopped nursing."

"How long did you nurse?" I ask.

She screws up her face. "Two weeks?"

"How did it go?"

"It was OK but a real pain, you know?"

I'm not sure if she means exasperating or uncomfortable. Lots of teenagers seem to like the idea of nursing but find it difficult in practice. It requires, particularly in the beginning, a considerable amount of dedication.

"Is that why you decided to stop?" I ask.

Lila turns her head and looks about the room. "I guess," she says.

I nod and continue with the exam. Her abdomen is flat, hard. Her cervix is closed tight as before, her uterus is back to its pre-pregnancy size, but her vaginal walls are more swollen than I'd expect.

"Lila, have you had intercourse yet?"

"Why?"

"I'm asking because your vagina looks swollen."

"Well," she says, rolling her eyes, "I suppose I *should* tell you I have a new boyfriend."

"Oh?" *Already?* A sinking feeling in the pit of my stomach. Maybe this is why she stopped nursing. "Tell me."

"James. He's *really* cute."

"How is he with Angel?"

"He likes her a lot." Lila sits up as soon as I'm finished. "Really," she says again. "He's nice. Why, you don't think I can get a decent boyfriend?"

I put my hand on Lila's arm. "I think you could have any man you set your heart on. I just don't want to hear about you being hurt again."

I help Lila to stand. "And I'm glad you got the Depo shot after you delivered. No more babies for now."

"No kidding," she says, and flees behind the curtain to dress, first chucking Angel on the cheek. The baby slumbers on, sucking her pacifier so it squeaks in and out of her mouth.

"He's eighteen," she shouts to me.

A new man. I wonder if James drives a long rusty car with a

throbbing loudspeaker. I wonder if he kills time in front of the bus stop on Main Street. Or maybe I have it all wrong. Maybe he has a job at Stop & Shop, a beige stock boy's shirt tucked into his chinos. Maybe he flirts with Lila when she comes in to buy formula.

"Well, I hope it works out for you," I call back.

I hope Lila gets her GED, gets a job, stays clean, and finds a young man who will love her for her tough spirit and sweet ways. I hope Angel has half a chance of entering kindergarten five or six years from now. It seems I'm always hoping *something* where Lila's concerned. And it's not just this particular girl and her baby. It's that there are so many Lilas.

She comes out from behind the curtain and picks up the infant carrier.

"I'll see you later. I already got an appointment for my next shot."

"Take care, Lila. I wake up at night and worry about you."

She doesn't know what to do when someone is nice to her, so she begins biting her finger.

Lila and I look at each other, and I see a fleeting response go by, changing her eyes for a moment. It's that same feeling I had months ago, when I wanted to hug her, to rock her like a mother.

Today, instead of closing down and running away, she holds my gaze.

In this precise second, I realize why I love what I do. In the clinic, as in life, it's the tiny, incremental steps that matter. The moments when we go forward with strength or make a good choice. The moments when we inch up one level, emotionally or physically, and then stay there, wobbly and teetering perhaps, but ready to keep going. This is one of those moments. And I'm here—what an honor this is—I'm right here holding Lila's hand.

She promises to bring me a picture of Angel. She lingers for a moment making small talk, then turns to leave, juggling the baby's carrier and crooning to her as they go into the hall. I follow as they make their way past the secretary's desk, past the waiting room and through the clinic door. When I return to the back room, there's a chart waiting, a new patient to see. This one is seventeen. Just pregnant. Blond and cheerful, a little chubby.

She wants her mother to stay in the room with her, the nurse tells me, to lend moral support and a hand to hold. During the exam, mother and daughter giggle together like girlfriends. As I leave the room, the mother pulls me aside and whispers in my ear: "I had my first baby when I was sixteen. And see? I did just fine."

Chapter 35

My very first experience as a patient, years before my encounter with Dr. Riley and long before I had a hysterectomy or a breast biopsy, came unexpectedly when I was twelve. Thrown from a horse during a riding lesson, I'd felt only minor aches and pains. Then, exactly seven days later, a thick stupor came over me. I couldn't raise my hand to bring a mouthful of soup to my mouth. I was too weak to stand, and suddenly I couldn't see out of one eye. The right side of my body felt hot and prickly; then it went numb.

My father rushed me to the hospital, where I stayed for days, diagnosed (my parents told me later, and I don't know how accurate their understanding was) with a blood clot that had been dislodged by the shock of my fall and was now traveling lazily through my brain, a small fragment that temporarily turned off various body functions as it meandered along. My parents were allowed to visit only one hour a day. It was the nurses who kept me company. Young, dressed in starched white uniforms with cupcake bonnets or winged caps that made them look like angels, they cajoled and mothered me. If I needed them, they appeared at my bedside instantly. I thought the polished hospital floor must be made of ice and the nurses must be skaters, whooshing quietly from room to room with thin sharp blades on their white shoes.

Their cool fingertips soothed my brow. Their breath was frosty peppermint.

It seemed to me that they loved all the patients in their ward, a ragged assortment of older women in flimsy striped gowns and me in my colorful pediatric nightie. During the day, we ladies sat propped up in our beds, waiting our turns to be bathed or slathered with lotion. The nurses' ministrations felt as real and as exhilarating to me as a gallop on the fastest horse. Their commitment to me felt as genuine as a parent's caring and concern, yet somehow more expert and less complicated. I could get mad at my nurses and know that they would return, uninjured. Best of all, in their presence, I didn't have to be brave.

Within a few weeks, I recovered totally, and soon I forgot about them. Even when my best friends began reading *Cherry Ames* or mimicking the nurses on popular TV shows, I remained firm. I never wanted to be a nurse. I wanted nothing to do with hospitals and needles and sickness. Instead, I would be an artist or a poet, someone who could be, I incorrectly imagined, less regimented and somehow protected from suffering. Years later, when I did gravitate toward nursing, fascinated by how we humans have the capacity to care for one another, body and soul, I wrote a poem about my first hospitalization and the young women who tended me. My evolving intrigue with caregiving, I realized, had begun with them. "I vowed I would always love their way," I wrote. "Fierce, physical."

Ever since, I've tried to care for my own patients with kindness and expertise. Some days I'm better at this than others. Like any caregiver, I can be overwhelmed by a hundred things: too many patients, too little staff, the aggravation and complexities of managed care, the limitations of poverty, the apathy of some of the patients themselves. Those days, I ask myself why I bother. Sometimes my own life interferes and my emotions ride very close to the surface because of a personal trauma: a parent's death, a child's distance, a grandchild's sudden severe illness. Then it's important for me to remember that although we share the same female body, its disturbances and events, I am separate from my patients and they from me. We have our own destinies to pursue and our individual tragedies to bear. I cannot save them, and saving them is not my job. But I can listen long and deep, my perception of their misfortunes sharpened by my own. I can forgive them almost anything and encourage them to start again because there is so much for which I have been forgiven.

On the best days, I come to work clear and balanced, alert to evidence of my patients' physical or emotional ills. My hands are gentle and sensitive, my brain is quick, my soul is open, my own house is in order. Then I become a woman who provides good care, fierce care, to other women, extraordinary women such as Lila, Eleanor, Joanna, Renée. The cast of characters in the clinic is forever changing, but they all stay in my memory.

Lila will be a part of my clinic world, I hope, for a long time. She will return every twelve weeks for her birth control shot and once a year for her annual exam. I don't know what time will bring, but I watch as Angel grows, plump and loved, and I see how Lila becomes a bit more mature with every visit. Eleanor's story, on the other hand, simply stopped.

When her new insurance card arrived, she came in to pick up her records and this time to say a real and final good-bye. Her frizzy hair was confined under a knit cap, and her hands were chapped from the cold, as if she'd been out for a vigorous walk. To me, she looked extremely healthy. Cheerful and formal, she shook hands with us all, me and Emily, Claire and Kate, Nina and Eric, Yanna and anyone else who happened to be in the clinic. As I stood talking with Eleanor, Lila and Angel almost collided with us.

Angel was awake, and Lila looked fresh and innocent.

"Hey, Lila," I said, and she beamed.

"Davis, where *were* you?" Lila said, waving a picture of Angel at me.

Eleanor's hands swooped to Angel's face. They tickled her cheeks and stroked her hair. "Oh my," she said, "what an adorable baby."

Lila angled Angel so Eleanor could get a better look.

"She's getting big," Lila said, and then turned to address me. "She eats like a piggy." She opened Angel's fuzzy jacket and popped the pacifier from her mouth.

"Say hello," she coaxed.

"Eleanor," I said, "this is Lila and Angel. Lila, this is Eleanor. She's a math teacher at the university."

Eleanor extended her hand to Lila, who looked baffled, then reached her hand out too.

"Ugh, I hate math," Lila said.

"That's OK," Eleanor replied. "I hate history." She asked if she could hold Angel. Lila looked at me as if to say "Can I trust this woman?" and then she gave Angel over into Eleanor's arms.

"Oh, how I'd love to have grandchildren," she said, and Lila, all her social graces on alert, asked, "You got any kids?"

Eleanor named her sons, and Lila whistled. "Wow," she said, "three!" and smiled at me. Every patient thinks I am hers alone. I think every patient is mine.

"I just came to give you this," Lila said and handed me a picture of Angel propped up on a squishy alphabet block with an assortment of toys behind her.

Eleanor and I, two women who would never again bear children, exclaimed over Angel's picture while our bodies, even without their uteruses, tingled with that odd, indefinable maternal zing. Lila, a young woman at the beginning of fertility's myriad and complex possibilities, stood back and blushed with pride.

I said good-bye to the three of them, and Eleanor and Lila strolled down the hall toward Kate's desk. "See you," they called to me, turning to wave. Lila and Angel walked off in one direction, Eleanor in another. It was the last time I saw her.

Joanna and Renée continue to visit the clinic. Joanna, whose graphic design business is flourishing, comes for her annual exams. Because we have shared such an intimate secret, we are often open and easy with each other; then we speak with our glances as well as our words. Other days, when her past is more burdensome, Joanna's conversation is edgy and strained. She's still in therapy, and I'm confident that she will survive. Perhaps not with the forward rush of the graceful gazelle she once reminded me of, but with the deliberate movements of a deer who picks her way delicately through the underbrush. The last time Joanna came to the clinic, she brought me photos of some of her paintings. A gift.

First there were the radiant oils from her student days in Florence, men and women backlit by sunlight glancing through a window. Like Giotto, she had traced a faint outline around each person to both separate and contain them. Then, abstract black-and-white geometric prints that looked spare and stark, lonely and desperate. Last, a few watercolors marked "These are the new ones" on the back. Vibrant washes of lemon, turquoise, azure, and violet, a field of wildflowers lush and bountiful.

"Thank you, Joanna," I said. I tucked her photos into my lab coat pocket, and later I took them home. They sit propped up on my bookshelf.

Renée visits more frequently. She can't afford the birth control pills she takes—*just in case,* she tells me—so I give her free samples every few months, although I'm sure the drug company would rather I wrote a prescription. Initially, Renée was the patient I liked least, the woman who came from the neighborhood most distant from mine. But Renée has become one of the patients I especially admire, the patient who continues to remind me that we *are* sisters, all of us, no matter our heritage or our destination. We walk the narrow edge between disability and physical health, between despair and strength. We share the ever-changing environment of the female body.

Renée has also taught me that although there may be many unalterable boundaries between me and my patients—among them age, culture, social circumstance, life experience, illness, and our separate roles of patient and caregiver—these divisions need not be barriers. I can reach beyond these differences to find our similarities, and that permits me to be, with any woman, a kind listener, a nonjudgmental counselor, and a skilled practitioner. Renée taught me not to fear being afraid when I face someone whose background is foreign to me, but to reach out anyway. Most of the time, that's all that's required.

I became reacquainted with Renée several months after she'd first left Marvin in the hospital, opting to place him temporarily in foster care. I was upstairs visiting Loretta after work when the automatic door to the NICU slid open, and there stood Renée. I looked, then looked again. She held Marvin nestled in her arms.

While I'd lost track of them, Loretta hadn't. She knew that Renée continued to visit Marvin in his foster home several times a week, even while she worked and saved and called every public assistance office to find out who would help her get an apartment. She attended all her counseling sessions and gave her urine tox screens willingly. She saved enough money for security and rent on a two-room walk-up apartment in an old Victorian house around the corner from the hospital. She bought a pile of toys and lived alone. All those months, she battled her demons until they became small and weak, and then, when the demons no longer called her name, she proved to Family Services that she was ready to take Marvin home.

"Renée!" we said.

"Ha, found you," Renée said. "Want to see Marvin?"

Marvin was seven months old, still smaller than most babies his age but catching up. He was dressed in a sailor's shirt and navy pants, and he had thick curly hair and long eyelashes. Every time we made him laugh, a single dimple appeared in his left cheek. When Renée talked to him, he didn't take his eyes from her face. This mother and baby were mutually enchanted.

"You know," Renée said, "I went every week and told him I was his mama. I told him that one day, for sure, I would take him home. And I did." Renée's grin was wide as her face. She didn't care that her hands were cracked from washing diapers and rinsing bottles. She didn't care that her day began at five and ended at midnight or later. Here she was, a woman with a family.

She took me aside.

"Is it OK with you if I come back to the clinic?" she asked.

"Of course," I replied, somewhat puzzled. I wondered why she thought it wouldn't be.

"I know I wasn't exactly your *favorite* patient," she said, swinging Marvin to her hip. "But I'm different now."

We stood together for several seconds. Same height, same tall and slender bodies, same moment in time. Every one of us goes through her changes, but I'd never accomplished anything so grand as Renée had.

"I believe you are," I replied. "And I'd be happy to see you."

Later, Loretta told me what she'd heard from Family Services. One of Renée's other three children had been adopted in infancy, but two remained in foster care. Renée had recently obtained permission to see them, an eight-year-old girl and a six-year-old boy. Once a week, she took Marvin and they went for a visit. It was possible, Loretta said, that if all went well, Family Services might let Renée take custody of her other two children as well.

"That woman started out with nothing," Loretta said. "Now look, she's ended up with almost everything."

This afternoon, Renée has an appointment with me for her annual Pap test and more birth control pills; maybe she'll have some good news. Joanna's name probably won't show up in the appointment book for my evening clinic for at least six months. In the meantime, when dusk comes and my late-day patients arrive or when I ask new patients about abuse, I think of Joanna and wonder how she's growing and changing. I think about Eleanor, too. Has she negotiated menopause with her usual good cheer? Will her cancer ever recur? Since I won't know, I can only wish for Eleanor not youth but the traits of youth: health, wonder, and the ability to exist in the moment while anticipating the future. Of course, Lila might show up at any time, surprising me. Lila, who gives me hope. Breathless and earnest, holding on to Angel, Lila arrives calling my name.

When I walk into the hallway, I hear the residents' laughter float out from the back room. We're especially busy today, and the nurses are determined to keep us moving. It's hard for me to believe that I've worked here almost ten years.

The secretary's desk is surrounded with patients, and I see that the waiting room is already full—women with their babies layered in blue and yellow blankets, young girls whose bodies are just beginning to awaken, and women whose bodies are, like mine, for now at peace. Our clinic is a small space, but its wonders are boundless.

I stand for a moment, watching.

Acknowledgments

Many thanks to the editors of the journals in which sections of this book, in earlier versions, first appeared: *Fetishes, So To Speak,* and *Witness.*

My gratitude to the Money for Women/Barbara Deming Memorial Fund for a grant that provided financial encouragement during my early work on this manuscript.

Appreciation also goes to Lori Negridge Allen, Silky Berger, Karla Bernstein, Meg Lindsay, Jean Sands, and Irene Sherlock for their indispensable suggestions; to Lynn Bernardini, R.N., my guide through the neonatal intensive care unit; and to Lester Silberman, M.D., who advised me about counseling patients regarding sexuality issues. My thanks to the clinic residents, past and present, for their friendship and technical advice, especially Elizabeth Kontarines, M.D., and Mary Beth Miller, M.D., and to the nurses and secretaries with whom I work, for their help and kindness.

I am indebted to my agent, the incredible Elyse Cheney, whose enthusiasm encouraged me, and to her assistants; to my editor, Courtney Hodell, whose wisdom midwifed this book into the world, and to Timothy Farrell, assistant editor; to Lauren Goldin, Sybil Pincus, Jynne Martin, and so many others at Random House, for their generous and expert attention.

Most of all, I thank my husband, Jon, whose love sustains me; my children, Lisa and Christopher, and their families, for their precious presence in my life; and my patients, for their bravery and trust.

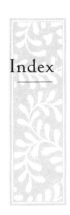

Index

About the Author

CORTNEY DAVIS is the author of two poetry collections, *The Body Flute* and *Details of Flesh,* and co-editor of *Between the Heartbeats: Poetry and Prose by Nurses.* She has received an NEA fellowship for her poetry, which appears in publications such as the *Journal of the American Medical Association, Hudson Review, Ontario Review,* and *Poetry.* An active participant in the field of literature and medicine, she often gives readings and workshops for health care professionals. Davis lives in Connecticut, where she is a nurse practitioner in women's health.

About the Type

This book was set in FF Celeste, a digital font that its designer, Chris Burke, classifies as a modern humanistic typeface. Celeste was influenced by Bodoni and Waldman, but the strokeweight contrast is less pronounced, making it more suitable for current digital typesetting and offset-printing techniques. The serifs tend to the triangular, and the italics harmonize well with the roman in tone and width. It is a robust and readable text face that is less stark and modular than many of the modern fonts and has many of the friendlier old-face features.